Escape from Diabetes

by

Precision Low-carb & Periodic Fasting

An Evidence-Based Guide

for Precision Diabetes Care

Dr. Younkuk Choi

Contents

Preface

When the hawk catches the pheasant, its natural instincts play a role, but its hunting ability honed by repeated training, sharp eyes, and accurate skill allows successful capture. Similarly, I was previously a hawk who was not good at catching pheasants when it came to diabetes, possibly because I was not thinking seriously enough about patients with diabetes. I mistakenly thought that modern medicine has addressed diabetes and told my patients to take the drugs prescribed.

However, as a physician who now treats patients and researches differences among humans, diseases, and food, I am a hawk who excels at catching pheasants; namely, intractable patients seeking help after losing hope from not finding any solutions at primary, secondary, and tertiary hospitals, despite stigmatizing myself as an unclassified quaternary hospital physician and recommending colleague and junior physicians to do the same when instructing them or sharing experiences. Despite catching pheasants well, this method of treating intractable diseases based on differences between individuals, diseases, and appropriate diet is not yet recognized. I have learned and am using the method of riding an airplane from meeting a great teacher in an age when everyone else is riding bicycles; thus, my methods are difficult for others to understand. It is an intermediate conclusion for which it is difficult to prove or receive recognition. I have spent considerable time describing an airplane in a world where people barely understand bicycles; however, there are many limitations.

I made up my mind that I should return to catching pheasants. As a physician who can resolve diabetes, which had been a missing link, I returned as a hawk that easily catches pheasants by supplementing the methods that were previously lacking. Now, I will stop harping about hawks and pheasants and get to the main point. Diabetes is not a disease and is certainly not an irreversible disease that requires management by taking drugs for the rest of your life. Do not believe that you are suffering a serious disease. There is absolutely no reason for you to despair or shed a tear. Diabetes is simply a symptom of overeating foods with fast rate of conversion to glucose. This is especially true for type 2 diabetes and its subtypes. Type 1 diabetes is a different world, though. Therefore, you can escape from diabetes by regularly eating small servings of foods that are suitable for you and have slow rates of conversion to glucose. Some people do not believe this is possible or are unsure even though they have experienced a complete escape. Therefore, this guide represents a compilation of the medical evidence and relevant knowledge regarding the phenomena that occur during escape from diabetes.

I would like to talk about my own past. I used to hastily eat three meals a day because I was pressed for time as I handled nearly 100 patients a day. I would often mix a small bowl of white rice with water or soup and gulp it down. The meal would take less than a minute. In midst of repetitive daily routines, my body had ballooned over several years. After gaining 30 kg, I found myself running out of breath and being uncomfortable whenever I had to walk uphill to return home after work. It was an emergency. My blood test results showed fatty liver and cholesterol, triglyceride, and glycated hemoglobin levels exceeding the cutoff values. I asked myself "Do I not exercise enough?" "I pick and eat foods that are beneficial for me, so why?"

"I don't eat a lot, so why is this happening?" I reviewed the foods I was eating with the help of my wife, who has a major in Oriental Rehabilitation Medicine. Fortunately, I received nutritional advice based on her experience with running an obesity clinic at the Oriental Medicine Hospital. Even then, I had lingering questions and few answers. I tried various experiments. While combining various knowledge, some of which I had forgotten since it had been a while, and making observations about body weight and meals, I noticed something strange. When I nervously compared my weight measured the day after eating a small bowl of rice as usual versus weight measured the day after eating a similar amount of ice cream, my weight had increased much more on the day after eating rice. Why did this happen? How could I weigh less after eating ice cream, which has much more calories due to its high milk fat content? Based on a few experiences, my experiment and research into food began in earnest. After 6 months, I had lost about 20 kg and my blood test values were all normal. This was the starting point of the precision diet for diabetes.

Subsequently, I had a new perspective on diabetic patients and realized the problems that are tangled in the background as well as the solutions to such problems. Diabetes can be overcome in more than 90% cases. I have become a hawk that excels at catching pheasants.

In addition to my own practice, I have shared these methods and knowledge with colleagues in the past decade to achieve amazing outcomes. However, because these methods have been limited to primary care, enough records could not be obtained to demonstrate sufficient evidence. I embarked on new efforts to overcome this situation. Digital technology is being integrated to conveniently record and collect information on meals and blood test results and assist in the implementation of a lifetime of health management with only lifestyle interventions and the consumption of beneficial foods by guiding patients to the finish line of escape from diabetes and weaning from drug therapy. These efforts are comprehensively referred to as precision diabetes care.

The information in this guide is designed to help guide patients through their journeys, from the beginning to when they may stumble or struggle. I am confident that this guide will be something to lean on when you stumble just before the finish line as doubts grow and your willpower flags.

Fortunately, physicians in various fields worldwide who have performed experiments almost identical to mine have been active for many years and I am elated to find that I am not alone. There is much debate and conflicting opinions regarding the adverse effects of implementing some programs without classifying people according to their differences and classifying foods according to such differences. I hope that this precision diabetes care guide adds wisdom to our understanding and integration of this global medical trend.

I extend my sincerest gratitude to my great master, Dr. Dowon Kuon, who enlightened me about differences among people and classification of food. Woojun Kuon, my mentor, who provided deep inspiration for the application of modern physiology and pathology; and Dr. Hyojeong Lee, my loving wife and colleague, who has been a positive hurdle to make me reflect whenever I faced new opportunities and challenges in my life.

Summer 2019

Younkuk Choi, MD (Korean Medicine)

Founding CEO of Precision Diabetes Care

R.TCMP/R.Ac. (ON, CANADA)

Dipl. O.M. (NCCAOM, USA)

I. Overview of diabetes

1. What is diabetes?

The term diabetes, short for diabetes mellitus, means excess sugar in the urine. Sugar refers to glucose, an element essential for brain and muscle function in the human body. However, for various reasons, the levels of glucose stored in the body may become excessive and be discharged through urine. Whatever its cause, diabetes is an indication of abnormally high glucose level in the body.

Despite its name, diabetes is not actually tested or diagnosed based on levels of sugar in the urine. Instead, hyperglycemia or diabetes are generally diagnosed based on the measurement of blood glucose levels, typically fasting blood sugar (FBS) 30 minutes before a meal or post-prandial 2-hour blood glucose (PP2). Glycated hemoglobin (HbA1c) level, which indicates the percentage of glucose bound to red blood cells (RBC), is also important.[1]

---

[1] For specific levels, refer to "Chapter II: Diabetes diagnosis and complications."

While polydipsia (increased thirst), polyphagia (increased appetite), and polyuria (frequent urination) are generally discussed as the three major symptoms of diabetes, diabetes is often detected by repeated manifestation and persistence of symptoms including excessive fatigue, dysthymia, sudden weight change, blurred vision, and frequent inflammation and delayed recovery or by chance during health examinations in patients with no perceived symptoms.

Type 2 diabetes is most commonly associated with obesity and is generally known to occur when the body is unable to secret insulin or cannot effectively use the insulin that has been secreted. Type 1 diabetes, the cause of which is difficult to determine, is known as a condition associated with very little or no insulin secretion. The other types of diabetes include gestational diabetes associated with pregnancy, monogenic diabetes that occurs rarely due to genetic defects in pancreatic beta cells, and other specific types[2] caused by other diseases or drugs.

____

[2] Refer to Diabetes Canada, 2018 Clinical Practice Guidelines,
http://guidelines.diabetes.ca/docs/CPG-2018-full-EN.pdf.

2. What is insulin and what role does it play?

Insulin[3] is a hormone secreted by pancreatic beta cells. It plays a role in transporting glucose in the blood to muscle, liver, and fat cells for use as energy. Most glucose in the body is supplied through the consumption and digestion of food. Glucose oversupply causes increased insulin secretion by the pancreas, whereby excess glucose in the blood is stored in the liver or fat cells. In contrast, during prolonged fasting, glucose stored in the liver and the whole body as fat is broken down by glycolysis as needed to maintain a consistent glucose level in the blood.[4]

---

[3] Refer to "Dr. Frederick Banting – Discovery of Insulin" on page 57 of Dr. Younkuk Choi's ECM Eyes, Current Medical News Commentaries.

[4] Refer to the National Institute of Diabetes and Digestive and Kidney Diseases (NIDDK) https://www.niddk.nih.gov/health-information

3. Why do people get diabetes?

The simplest and most accurate answer to this question is "eating too much." This answer applies to most cases of type 2 and gestational diabetes. Of course, this does not include type 1 and rare types of diabetes. Anyone who does not want to read further and throw away this book after reading this answer should give up on escaping from diabetes. Overeating is the direct cause of type 2 diabetes; while it has been attributed to over 85% of cases, empirical assessments in actual clinical settings suggest that the rate is much higher than 90%. Insulin secretion increases as a normal response to the explosive increase in glucose levels in the body due to overeating. Continued overeating eventually reaches a point at which insulin can no longer respond normally and process glucose. Accordingly, blood insulin levels become hyperinsulinemic and insulin does not function properly; thus, type 2 diabetes is defined as the condition in which the body is not able to properly use insulin present in the body. It does not arise from the pancreas not secreting enough insulin or due to secretion dysfunction for unknown reasons, as is the perception in modern medicine. The pancreas and insulin continue to work hard but the biggest problem is the continued supply of glucose beyond the level that can be handled[5]. Awareness of this problem is the start of escaping from diabetes.

---

[5] For more detailed mechanistic opinions, refer to the video by Dr. Jason Fung, titled "Understanding and treating Type 2 diabetes" at https://www.dietdoctor.com. This opinion is consistent with the lengthy clinical and research experiences of the author. However, since there are major differences in coping methods, refer to "Chapter IV: Precision diet for diabetes" for further details.

4. Why is diabetes comorbid with symptoms of metabolic syndrome such as fatty liver, hypertriglyceridemia, hypercholesterolemia, obesity, and hypertension?

Excessive glucose introduced into the body from overeating is primarily stored on the liver surface as fat by the actions of insulin. However, continued excessive glucose intake causes fat accumulated on the liver surface to exceed the normal range. In such cases, ultrasonographic examination can confirm the diagnosis of fatty liver. If the liver surface is likened to a storage space, it is a primary storage space that can store very little. In contrast, fat cells found throughout the body represent a very large secondary storage space whose size and volume continue to increase like a soap bubble from absorbing glucose. Consequently, the body gradually becomes overweight, eventually leading to obesity. This phenomenon is not readily recognized since there are no perceived symptoms other than continued weight gain and elevated blood pressure (BP). Fat that is not stored roams freely in blood vessels, causing elevated blood triglyceride (TG) level.

Moreover, fat binds with proteins to cause decreased high-density lipoprotein (HDL) level and increased low-density lipoprotein (LDL) and very-low-density lipoprotein (VLDL) levels in the blood or is deposited on vessel walls[6]. At this stage, there are still no superficial symptoms. If such situations are not recognized and overeating or binge eating continue, increased levels of glucose that has not yet been or can no longer be converted to fat and cannot bind with other factors may cause hyperglycemia (diabetes). These processes may appear sequentially or simultaneously and, if they persist, may cause a variety of complex complications.

---

[6] Marc-Andre Cornier, Dana Dabelea, Teri L. Hernandez, Rachel C. Lindstrom, Amy J. Steig, Nicole R. Stob, Rachael E. Van Pelt, Hong Wang, Robert H. Eckel, "The Metabolic Syndrome", Endocrine Reviews, vol. 29, Issue 7, Dec. 1, 2008, pp. 777–822

5. What are the criteria for overeating?

Patients with type 2 diabetes often do not agree that their current amount and method of food intake is overeating. This is due to a lack of awareness about the definition of overeating. Overeating is a relative concept. People often mistakenly believe they are not overeating because they eat relatively less than those around them. Moreover, light eating, which is the opposite of overeating, has no set values such as how many grams should be consumed in a day. However, the state of hyperglycemia is the output of a simple mathematical calculation, which indicates that the amount of glucose introduced into and digested by the body, by whatever reason and means, is more than the amount of glucose used by the brain and muscles.

If you cannot answer positively to the following three scenarios, you should consider yourself an overeater. Firstly, are you hungry enough before the next meal? After a meal, you should feel hungry for at least 30 minutes to an hour before the next meal to the point of your stomach growling no matter how small the previous meal and how active you were. If this is not the case and you are eating your next meal just because it is mealtime, then this is an indication that you are overeating. Secondly, do you eat regular meals? Regular meals mean a consistent glucose intake. The human body is well trained for such regularity. The body stores only a minimal amount in preparation for the worst-case scenario and regularly discards any surplus. In contrast, the body is vulnerable to irregularity but is well prepared for these instances. Because it is difficult to anticipate the next meal, the body stores little when a small amount is consumed and much more when larger amounts are consumed, storing all without discarding it in preparation for the next extreme hunger situation. Accordingly, large amounts of fat are stored in the body to keep up with overeating. Accordingly, people who eat small portions irregularly store more fat in their bodies than those who regularly eat larger portions. Together with the frustration of gaining weight despite being a light eater, the persistence of this eating pattern may lead to metabolic diseases including diabetes. Thirdly, do grains[7] comprise

---

[7] Grains were used as an example of a food group with high glycemic index (GI) and glycemic load (GL). Refer to "Chapter IV: Precision diet for diabetes" for further explanation.

less than approximately one-quarter of a single meal? Grains have the fastest rate of conversion to glucose inside the body. Despite accounting for only 2% of total body weight, the brain uses 20% of glucose introduced into the body,[8] with the remaining glucose used by the muscles. Compared to the past, modern humans use their brains more than their muscles. Recommended dietary intakes with grains accounting for half or more of daily consumption remain suitable for farming and hunting situations, as well as physical laborers, athletes, and highly active children with high muscle use and high activity levels. However, this recommended intake is not suitable for the daily activities of modern humans. Grain intake exceeding one-quarter of a single meal indicates excessive glucose consumption; in modern humans who only move their fingers in front of a computer as their daily activity, this represents overeating.

---

[8] Mergenthaler, Philipp et al. "Sugar for the brain: the role of glucose in physiological and pathological brain function." Trends in neurosciences vol. 36,10 (2013): 587-97.

6. Is diabetes inherited?

Evidence of the inheritance or genetic associations of diabetes is weak[9]. It is safe to assume that type 2 diabetes has no genetic associations. In other words, it is not a congenital disease. The real culprit is acquired dietary habits. Because family members have similar dietary habits, diabetes often appears to have a genetic link. However, this is not an irreversible problem; it can be reversed by correcting poor dietary habits that cause diabetes, obesity, and metabolic syndrome[10]. For now, at least, you should not be concerned about family history or genetics. Proper use and practice of the recommendations in this guide will provide experience and confidence that there are also no such concerns in the future.

---

[9] Pay attention to the conclusion derived by Valeriya Lyssenko and Markku Laakso in their article "Genetic Screening for the Risk of Type 2 Diabetes", Diabetes Care, Aug. 2013, 36 (Supplement 2) S120-S126, published by the American Diabetes Association (ADA) – *"Genetic testing for the prediction of type 2 diabetes in high risk individuals is currently of little value in clinical practice."*

[10] The utmost priority should be placed on dietary habits and their importance relative to other lifestyle changes and exercise. Priorities #1–5 are dietary habits and exercise could be considered priority #6. Refer to "Chapter IV: Precision diet for diabetes" for further details.

7. Are certain people or lifestyle habits more prone to diabetes?

Many people eat a lot and continuously, eat little but very irregularly, or have dietary habits such as rushing to take a quick meal consisting mostly of carbohydrates such as rice, noodles, ramen, hamburger, or sandwiches. However, when such lifestyles become habit, there is no way to avoid diabetes and other conditions. Before the onset of diabetes, obesity and a series of metabolic syndrome symptoms, including hypertension, fatty liver, hypercholesterolemia, and hypertriglyceridemia, appear. This also applies to people who cannot remember the last time they performed any kind of cardiovascular or muscle exercise. People sometimes place too much importance on exercise; however, not getting enough exercise is not a direct cause of diabetes. Type 2 diabetes cannot be avoided by anyone without a diet consisting of precise nutritional proportions based on their meal amount and regularity, activity level, and metabolic rate. Conversely, diabetes can be easily escaped with dietary correction. This is the easiest, and at the same time, the hardest part.

Another important part is that some factors related to the development of diabetes could be attributed to differences among individuals. Some people with good digestion and appetite always overeat, whereas some people eat just enough to survive with no interest in food or who find eating to be a burdensome process. People with overflowing appetite could certainly avoid diabetes if they exercise self-control, but it would obviously be difficult if they simply followed their instincts. For the most part, people with little interest in food tend to have a very low probability of being overweight or developing diabetes.

Rarely, there are differences based on types of food. Not only type 2 but also type 1 diabetes can result when people who should eat meat instead enjoy being vegetarians or people who should avoid chicken or spicy food constantly eat such foods.

Typically, people who are unable to control their consumption of foods that cause an explosive increase in glucose levels are most prone to developing diabetes. However, people who fail to qualitatively differentiate foods that are good or bad for them could also develop type 1 diabetes or extremely rare type of diabetes due to the long-term disruption of the hormonal and immune systems.

8. Can you get diabetes from eating too much sugar? What about stevia, xylitol, honey, and syrup?

If you lean toward "much" (quantity of sugar), the answer would be "Yes," whereas if you lean toward "sugar" (quality itself), the answer would be "No." Not only sugar, but the consumption of too much of any food can cause diabetes. Sugar itself is not guilty. In the past, sugar was used as medicine or a luxury good in the East and West and had beneficial effects in some people. The sugar that we typically eat is sucrose refined from sugar cane. Sucrose is composed of glucose linked to fructose. Along with maltose (glucose-glucose) and lactose (glucose-galactose), they are classified as disaccharides. However, the cells in our body are interested only in the monosaccharides glucose and fructose, which are broken down by intestinal enzymes. Glucose is easily converted to energy; however, fructose can only be converted to energy by liver cells. Consequently, large quantities of fructose burdens the liver to convert fructose to energy. Liquid fructose (high-fructose corn syrup) is very inexpensive and tastes sweeter taste than glucose. The food industry uses liquid fructose in a variety of ways; as a result, its consumption is skyrocketing. This increased consumption is closely associated with the advent of diabetes and metabolic syndrome as major health issues[11]. Stevia, which is used in small amounts due to its strong sweet taste, or xylitol, which is not converted to glucose, are alternatives for diabetic patients; however, there are few reasons for their use in the first place. Honey or syrups also do not cause diabetes on their own. You simply need to be cautious about whether something is appropriate and control intake.

The reason for explaining these somewhat complicated actions to understand the differences in the effects of glucose (a monosaccharide) and sugar (a disaccharide) is that no matter the type of sugar, excessive intake is problematic. However, accurate differentiation is possible only by recognizing the variations in response due to differences among individuals and in the characteristics of

---

[11] Refer to Ferris Jabr, "Is Sugar Really Toxic? Sifting through the Evidence", Scientific American, Jul. 15, 2013, https://blogs.scientificamerican.com/brainwaves/is-sugar-really-toxic-sifting-through-the-evidence/

these types of sugars. People who were born with strong liver function could achieve health improvement from suppressing liver function by consuming appropriate amounts of sugar and even liquid fructose. In contrast, for people who born with weak liver function, any substance other than glucose, which converts easily to energy without burdening the liver, cannot produce good results.

Therefore, both quantitative problems and qualitative characteristics must be considered for proper approaches to sugar, other types of saccharides, diabetes, metabolic syndrome, and even overall health issues.

9. What about exclusive diets consisting of health supplements or specific foods known to be good for diabetes?

Type 2 diabetes starts from overeating. In particular, the main culprit is the excessive consumption of food with high carbohydrate content. You cannot prevent a cup of water from overflowing by adding something to the cup. No more water must be poured. It is that simple. Therefore, there is no such thing as a food that is good for diabetes. The right answer is that whatever the food may be, it must be reduced or eliminated when diabetes is involved.

However, type 1 diabetes is different. Unlike type 2 diabetes, in which excessive quantities of food are the problem, autoimmune problems caused by dysfunction in qualitative characteristics are suspected to cause type 1 diabetes. This is a topic that requires further research. Even in such cases, the priority should be to find the types of food that are suitable for you. Even if there are health supplements or foods with enough proof of hypoglycemic effect, they must be checked to make sure they are suitable for you. If they are not suitable for you, the effects will soon become adverse events. No health supplements or specific foods have demonstrated clear evidence of curing diabetes. In fact, there are more cases of people getting further away from escaping from diabetes due to increased sugar levels from the consumption health supplements full of starches based on false information or from eating food harmful to them for their reported effects in lowering blood sugar level.

10. Could eating mostly brown rice or mixed grains be harmful?

Shells of grains consist mostly of fiber. The fiber in the outer shell of brown rice plays a role in digesting carbohydrates and slowing the rate of glucose conversion. Mixed grains generally have slower glucose conversion than that for white rice. However, consuming high percentages of grains, including brown rice and mixed grains, in all meals could be problematic when diabetes is involved. Sometimes, people are duped into believing that brown rice is good for diabetes and eat brown rice with every meal. Insisting on only brown rice without any meat or vegetables could be harmful to someone with diabetes. They will never escape from diabetes. Doing so could often cause digestive problems from eating food that is not suitable for them. If brown rice or a specific grain is suitable, keeping the percentage of such grains within 20% of the diet could be beneficial.

11. Is diabetes a disease from which it is impossible to recover?

In most patients with type 2 diabetes (over 90%), recovery is possible regardless of the extended use of medications or insulin injections. The key is proper diet, meaning light eating with precise control over the amount, eating regularly, and strictly adhering to proportions. For long-term effects, you must differentiate the types of foods that are right for you and eat them accordingly. Type 1 diabetes remains incurable in most cases. However, the dietary regimen for type 2 diabetes could significantly reduce the amount of insulin used.

The concept of curing diabetes by changing one's diet without drugs or insulin has been around for a while but it has gained recognition among physicians and patients worldwide in the past decade. Evidence from actual treatment cases and study results[12] continue to be published.

---

[12] Athinarayanan SJ, Adams RN, Hallberg SJ, et al., "Long-term effects of a novel continuous remote care intervention including nutritional ketosis for the management of type 2 diabetes: a 2-year non-randomized clinical trial", Frontiers in Endocrinology, 2019; 10:348.

The American Diabetes Association (ADA) defined diabetes as "a progressive disease requiring more medicine over time"[13]. However, Dr. Sarah Hallberg from the US claimed in her TED lecture that reversing type 2 diabetes should start with ignoring the ADA guidelines and drug use should be discontinued for treatment by diet[14]. Dr. Jason Fung from Canada and Dr. Andreas Eenfeldt from Sweden have joined efforts to publicize how dietary therapy can reverse diabetes. The national healthcare system in England has implemented a cutting-edge care program to reverse diabetes through diet[15]. The Royal Australian College of General Practitioners (RACGP), the largest such organization in Australia, has also issued guidelines for dietary therapy for type 2 diabetes[16]. Thus, type 2 diabetes is reversible with dietary therapy.

Refer to latest studies, including Ronald Scweizer, Ron Raa, "Concerns regarding the case of a man with newly diagnosed NIDDM", AJGP, vol.48, no. 6, Jun. 2019; 345

[13] For the original, refer to "Diabetes is a progressive disease requiring more medicine over time" and YouTube video in citation 14 below

[14] Refer to YouTube video titled "Reversing Type 2 diabetes starts with ignoring the guidelines", "Stop using medicine to treat food", https://www.youtube.com/watch?v=da1vvigy5tQ

[15] Nicholas Fearn , "Meet The Tech Company Looking To Reverse Type 2 Diabetes In 10 Million People", Forbes, Jan. 24, 2019

One thing to keep in mind and be cautious of is the rate of recovery. Recovery can be achieved but the rate is slow in patients who have relied on drugs and insulin for decades without reversing type 2 diabetes. Patients must anticipate the results to appear within months to years and remain patient. Moreover, patients need to understand that the rate of recovery may be very slow for those who have been on continuous drug therapy, especially sulfonylurea, even if for a short time.

---

[16] The Royal Austrian College of General Practitioners, "General practice management of type 2 diabetes 2016-2018", East Melbourne, Vic: RACGP, 2016., p.34.

12.   Is regeneration possible if the pancreas has almost ceased functioning due to prolonged drug therapy and having diabetes for a long time?

Some reports have indicated the beneficial effects of fasting and fasting-mimicking diet (FMD). Specifically, a famous study by Professor Valter Longo from the University of Southern California in the US reported the restoration of a damaged pancreas. He experimentally demonstrated the process by which mice placed under FMD were able to regain normal blood sugar regulation function through the regeneration of damaged pancreatic beta cells to secrete insulin[17].

What about humans? Based on my lengthy clinical experience, I believe that these experimental results could be applied to humans. My experience suggests that recovery is impossible in approximately 10% of patients with type 2 diabetes. Some of these cases may include patients with long-term use of the anti-diabetic drug sulfonylurea[18], while the reason is difficult to determine in

---

[17] Cheng, Chia-Wei et al. "Fasting-mimicking diet promotes Ngn3-driven β-cell regeneration to reverse diabetes", Cell, vol. 168, Issue 5, 775 - 788. e12

very few cases. However, escape from diabetes is possible in most cases, regardless of the length of anti-diabetic drug or insulin use. Accordingly, intensive application of a precision diet for diabetes in the initial stage, followed by a transition to standard light eating after enough time has passed, has shown no sudden increase in sugar levels. Moreover, the stable condition is maintained. Since these results were achieved in clinical practice without anti-diabetic drug or insulin use, it was believed that the pancreas, which had been almost completely nonfunctional, had recovered. At the cellular level, the results could also be interpreted as the regeneration of cells from cell death.

---

[18] Refer to "Chapter III: Treatment of diabetes" for the specific reasons.

13. How is diabetes correlated with obesity?

"Diabesity," combining dia- from diabetes and -besity from obesity, is a new term that has been used for several years in association with type 2 diabetes. Excessive glucose intake increases the size of fat cells throughout the body. Consequently, the size increases indiscriminately in areas that typically have high fat distribution, including the visceral area, thighs, hips, and cheeks. Until the excessive glucose intake stops, most cases of type 2 diabetes are comorbid with obesity. Childhood obesity involves increases in both fat cell size and number, whereas adult obesity involves only an increase in the size of fat cells. Therefore, overeating habits during childhood have negative health effects, including diabetes, throughout life.

Weight gain is an important predictor of diabetes. Obesity is associated with various diseases, including diabetes, metabolic disorders, and even cancer[19]. However, with respect to the magnitude of weight gain that could cause

[19] National Institute of Diabetes and Digestive and Kidney Diseases(NIDDK), "Health Risks of Being Overweight", https://www.niddk.nih.gov/health-information

medical problems, there are conflicting opinions based on various standards, including body mass index (BMI), waist-to-hip ratio, and 5–10% of standard body weight. Based on my clinical experience, a weight gain exceeding 10% of the body weight maintained during a 10-year period when a person was healthiest crosses the line into risky territory. Accordingly, the goal of weight control should also be a weight loss of 10% as a shortcut to escape from type 2 diabetes.

Precision diets for diabetes, as the name indicates, were designed precisely to escape from diabetes; however, due to the comorbidity of obesity in patients with type 2 diabetes, the diets are also effective for escaping from obesity.

14. What is the reason behind the explosive increase in diabetes among semi-developed and Asian countries, excluding some advanced countries?

In 2016, the World Health Organization (WHO) issued a report recommending aggressive measures for patients with diabetes, the number of which increased four-fold since 1980, mostly in developing countries[20]. Excessive glucose intake by over and binge eating is generally considered the cause of diabetes. However, it is somewhat puzzling to find that diabetes has become a greater problem in developing countries with less abundance of food.

A similar phenomenon is often seen in clinical practice. Many affluent people eat small portions of high-quality, balanced meals. They are not lazy about exercising and receive timely health screenings while also having leisure time. Thus, they have a low likelihood of facing problems associated with overeating, such as diabetes or obesity. In contrast, people with economic difficulties or no leisure time have a very high likelihood of developing diabetes.

---

[20] WHO, "Global report on diabetes", 2016.

They often binge eat, eat irregularly, or hastily eat foods with high glycemic index (GI).

This phenomenon is the same at the personal and national levels. It applies to countries experiencing economic development for the past 40 years. It is also similar in Asian countries where farming, which demands day-long labor, is the main industry. Another reason is the continuation of cultures that consider rice with high GI to be the main staple food in countries with rapid economic development. With mechanization of farming and use of computer control devices, muscle use has decreased drastically. Accordingly, since consumption of glucose introduced into the body is significantly reduced, it accumulates as fat in our body. In very poor countries, this increase could be attributed aid packages from advanced countries comprised primarily of surplus crops such as corn and flour. The report reflects the consequences of the change from staple foods consisting of small amounts of proteins obtained from hunting as well as rough grains to those containing highly refined grains with high GI.

II. Diabetes diagnosis and complications

1. What are the diagnostic criteria for diabetes?

Diabetes is often difficult to detect by symptoms alone. It is commonly diagnosed from levels exceeding the normal ranges in regular health screening. FBS and HbA1c are the major indicators. FBS should be measured after a fast of least 8 hours, meaning 30 minutes before breakfast. In addition, PP2 measured 120 minutes after the start of meal and oral glucose tolerance test (OGTT) to measure blood glucose levels two hours post-prandial following a 75-g oral glucose load can be used for reference. Generally, HbA1c is measured by a blood test performed in a hospital, clinic, or health center[21], while FBS and PP2 are commonly measured using self-monitoring glucometers.

The diagnostic criteria for diabetes include the items described above. However, because the test items, diagnostic criteria, and units of value are not consistent worldwide, these values and criteria need to be closely

---

[21] At-home A1C self-check kits have recently become available.

examined. The diagnostic criteria for diabetes used in South Korea, US, and Canada are shown below:

South Korea

Normal values

1) Fasting plasma glucose (FPG): <100 mg/dL,

2) 2-h PG during 75 g OGTT: <140 mg/dL

Prediabetes (diabetes high-risk group) is divided into different types:

1) Impaired fasting glucose (IFG): FPG 100–125 mg/dL,

2) Impaired glucose tolerance (IGT): 2-h PG 75 g OGTT 140–199 mg/dL,

3) Prediabetes (high risk for diabetes): HbA1c 5.7–6.4%

Diabetes is defined as;

1) HbA1c ≥6.5%, or

2) FPG ≥126 mg/dL, or

3) 2-h PG 75 g OGTT ≥200 mg/dL,

4) Traditional symptoms of diabetes (polyuria, polydipsia, and unexplained weight loss) and random plasma glucose (RPG) ≥200 mg/dL[22].

US

Normal values

1) FPG: <100 mg/dL

2) 2-h PG during OGTT <140 mg/dL

3) HbA1c <5.7%

Prediabetes is defined as;

1) FPG 100–125 mg/dL (5.6 –6.9 mmol/L),

2) 2-h PG during OGTT 140–199 mg/dL (7.8–11.0 mmol/L),

3) HbA1c 5.7–6.4 % (39–47 mmol/mol)

Diabetes is defined as;

---

[22] Korean Diabetes Association, http://www.diabetes.or.kr, refer to "2019 Diabetes Treatment Guidelines"

1) FPG ≥126 mg/dL (7.0 mmol/L),

2) 2-h PG during OGTT ≥200 mg/dL (11.1 mmol/L),

3) Random or casual plasma glucose ≥200 mg/dL (11.1 mmol/L) in patients with hyperglycemic symptoms,

4) HbA1c ≥6.5% (48 mmol/mol)[23].

Canada

Normal values

FPG <5.6 mmol/L and/or HbA1C <5.5%

At risk is defined as;

FPG of 5.6–6.0 mmol/L and/or HbA1c of 5.5–5.9%

Prediabetes is defined as;

FPG of 6.1–6.9 mmol/L and/or HbA1c of 6.0–6.4%

---

[23] American Diabetes Association, http://www.diabetes.org, "2. Classification and Diagnosis of Diabetes: Standards of Medical Care in Diabetes—2019 American Diabetes Association Diabetes Care", Jan. 2019; 42 (Supplement 1): S13-S28.

Diabetes is defined as;

FPG $\geq$ 7.0 mmol/L and/or HbA1c $\geq$ 6.5%[24].

For clarity, the information is organized in the table below. However, the following three values should remembered.

- FBS[25] $\geq$ 126 mg/dL (7.0 mmol/L),

- PP2 $\geq$ 200 mg/dL (11.1 mmol/L),

- HbA1c $\geq$ 6.5% as the criteria used for the diagnosis of **diabetes**.

However, depending on the situation, the management targets may not be consistent with these values in patients diagnosed with diabetes based on these criteria. In

---

[24] Diabetes Canada Clinical Practice Guidelines Expert Committee, "Diabetes Canada 2018 Clinical Practice Guidelines for the Prevention and Management of Diabetes in Canada", Can J Diabetes. 2018;42(Suppl 1):S1-S325.

[25] Fasting blood sugar and fasting plasma glucose could be considered to have the same meaning.

particular, there is controversy regarding the diabetes diagnostic criterion for HbA1c of ≥6.5% and the common standard of ≤7% as the management target in the US and Canada, which will be explained in detail in "What is the target HbA1c value?"

	US	Canada	South Korea
Normal	FPG < 100 mg/dL	FPG < 5.6 mmol/L	FPG < 100 mg/dL
	2-h PG during OGTT < 140 mg/dL	and/or	2-h PG during 75 g OGTT: <140 mg/dL
	HbA1c < 5.7 %	HbA1c < 5.5 %	

	US	Canada	South Korea
At risk		FPG of 5.6–6.0 mmol/L and/or HbA1c of 5.5–5.9%	1) Impaired fasting glucose (IFG): FPG 100–125 mg/dL, 2) Impaired glucose tolerance (IGT): 2-h PG 75 g OGTT

	US	Canada	South Korea
Prediabetes	1) FPG 100–125 mg/dL (5.6 –6.9 mmol/L), 2) 2-h PG during OGTT 140–199 mg/dL (7.8–11.0 mmol/L), 3) HbA1c 5.7–6.4 % (39–47 mmol/mol)	FPG of 6.1–6.9 mmol/L and/or HbA1c of 6.0–6.4%	140–199 mg/dL, 3) Prediabetes (high risk for diabetes): HbA1c 5.7–6.4%

	US	Canada	South Korea
Diabetes	1) FPG ≥126 mg/dL (7.0 mmol/L) 2) 2-h PG during OGTT ≥200 mg/dL (11.1 mmol/L), 3) Random or casual plasma glucose ≥200 mg/dL (11.1 mmol/L) in patients with hyperglycemic symptoms	FPG ≥7.0 mmol/L and/or HbA1c ≥6.5%	1) HbA1c ≥6.5% or 2) FPG ≥126 mg/dL or 3) 2-h PG 75 g OGTT ≥200 mg/dL 4) Traditional symptoms of diabetes (polyuria, polydipsia, and

	4) HbA1c ≥6.5% (48 mmol/mol)		weight loss) and random plasma glucose (RPG) ≥200 mg/dL

2. What is prediabetes?

The concept known as prediabetes, or prediabetic stage, is fraught with controversy[26]. While there are various claims, actual experience in clinical practice indicates that there is no need for concern based on values that qualify as prediabetes. In other words, there are many cases in which unnecessary preventive measures, such as drug prescription, are taken at prediabetic stage by mentioning the possibility of developing diabetes from prediabetes. However, there is absolutely no reason for such measures. Because diabetes develops from continued overeating, prediabetes should be considered a warning sign to reduce meal portions, examine dietary habits, and review lifestyle. Prediabetes should not be mistaken as a form of disease. Just as its name indicates, it is merely a pre-stage. However, it does require caution.

---

[26] Refer to the original article from *The New York Times*, titled "You're 'Prediabetic'? Join the Club" published on Dec.16, 2016 and the commentary on this article in Dr. Younkuk Choi's ECM Eyes, Current Medical News Commentaries.

3. Should blood sugar levels be checked daily?

Blood sugar levels should be measured daily when FBS or HbA1c levels are outside the normal ranges and require management. While cumbersome, one set each of FBS and PP2 needs to be measured every day for the time being. It is best to measure FBS after waking in the morning and before breakfast. Moreover, because modern people are busy during the afternoon, it is difficult to check PP2. Therefore, the PP2 check can be skipped during the day. It is often more convenient to measure PP2 after dinner. In most cases, measurement of blood sugar levels involves pricking one's own finger to sample blood, which makes it difficult to continue. However, it is absolutely necessary to monitor changes in blood sugar levels in the early stage of dietary management. Moreover, it is also necessary for monitoring and managing changes when drug administration is reduced or discontinued.

However, you should have hope since this is not something that you need to do throughout your entire life. Anyone who checks his or her blood sugar level every day for as little as three months often knows when to stop or realizes when a near-cure state has been reached. In fact, blood sugar levels often reach the normal range immediately or within a few days after starting precision diet for diabetes. While this may be hard to believe, it may be meaningful to measure blood sugar level every day to see the dramatic changes with your own eyes. Despite the pain of having to prick yourself, you will definitely have hope.

Fortunately, continuous glucose monitoring (CGM) devices[27] are becoming more available. The price of these devices is still a hurdle but putting up with the pain from a needle prick once every 7–14 days or 2–4 times a month enables blood sugar level to be checked automatically for 24 hours. This is more convenient than having to prick yourself twice daily. The price of these devices is expected to drop as they become more readily available.

---

[27] Dexcom , Abbott and other companies are competitively introducing their own CGM products.

4. For how long should blood sugar levels be checked?

Blood sugar levels should be checked from the time when precision diabetes care is started until FBS and HbA1c levels drop to the target ranges to allow observation of the process of blood sugar decreases due to the effects of dietary therapy and surveillance for unexpected adverse effects or hypoglycemia from an excessive drop in blood sugar level due to anti-diabetic drug use. At the same time, this measurement also provides motivation demonstrating firsthand how dietary management can effectively lower blood sugar levels without drugs or injections. It certainly has enough value as a guide in going from despair to hope of escaping from diabetes. Isn't the pain of pricking yourself to draw blood for a certain period worthwhile if it allows you to have hope for a complete recovery?

In the beginning stage, the frequency could be set to every day or at least three times a week as prescribed by the primary physician. Once the levels are managed within their normal ranges, checking for about one more month is recommended. After that, you do not need to have your finger pricked. You just need to manage your weight. Because type 2 diabetes is closely linked to obesity and overweight, there is no reason to draw blood every day once blood sugar levels have normalized. Measuring your weight every day and checking your HbA1c once every three months should be enough. A kit for self-measurement of HbA1c[28] level is also available.

---

[28] A1C Now Plus from PTS Diagnostics. https://ptsdiagnostics.com/.

5. Is it important to check body weight together with blood sugar level?

Type 2 diabetes is directly linked to being overweight or obesity, to the point of being called diabesity[29]. Therefore, stabilization of blood sugar level and body weight are closely correlated. In other words, they increase and decrease together. Consequently, when checking blood sugar level, always check body weight. As blood sugar levels drop, the body weight will also decrease and your body will feel much lighter. Any esthetic benefit will be a bonus. In addition, you may also gain psychological benefits such as self-confidence.

Once the blood sugar level is maintained and managed within the normal range, it is fine to check only the body weight every day. This can be a tool that allows you to escape from the agony of having to prick your finger to draw blood. It is the easiest and most effective method of managing the stabilized situation.

---

[29] Refer to "Chapter I-13. How is diabetes correlated with obesity?"

6. When is the best time to check body weight?

Many people are fearful of measuring their body weight or showing their results to others. It is understandable. However, covering up a problem could lead to an even bigger problem. Is there anything simpler and easier in daily life than measuring your body weight? There is nothing more cost-effective than making that simple act a daily ritual. It is not simply for diabetes, obesity, and metabolic disorders. Managing body weight is a simple yet an important factor in serious diseases such as cancer.

Make it a habit to weigh yourself every morning after the first urination as soon as you wake up. There is no need for difficult preparations or expensive measurement devices. A simple analog scale is enough and may be more accurate than a digital scale. Because a digital scale shows an exact number, people often react too sensitively to changes. However, do not become obsessed with the numbers themselves; instead, look at the overall trend. Unless you are experimenting, do not weigh yourself multiple times during the same day. Weighing yourself only once – at the same time immediately after waking, under the same conditions – and keeping a record of the results are recommended.

7. What are the differences between FBS and PP2? Why does PP2 decrease easily but FBS does not or increases after lengthy fasting?

Daily FBS and PP2 measurements are not highly reliable indicators for diabetes identification and diagnosis. However, they play an important role in monitoring and managing daily trends. Therefore, there is no need to be excited or distraught over these indicators. In particular, PP2 fluctuates quite a bit, increasing after eating just a little and quickly decreasing after exercise. Therefore, it would be a mistake to believe that the blood sugar level has stabilized based on a slight drop in PP2. Generally, PP2 drops quickly as soon as dieting starts. Occasionally, people fear elevated blood sugar levels after a meal. This is a wrong perception. Sometimes, people worry that their blood sugar level is too high at 30 minutes or one hour after meals. PP2 is like fireworks, in which glucose levels explode (peak) shortly after consumption before descending immediately thereafter. After reaching the peak value, it should drop to below 200 mg/dL (11.1 mmol/L) after about two hours. Measurement at 30 minutes or an hour would inevitably be much higher. A lack of high blood sugar level immediately after a meal would indicate a serious problem such as nutrients not being absorbed by the small intestines.

In contrast, FBS is a more reliable marker than PP2. FBS and HbA1c values are typically considered important for diagnostics and observation. FBS indicates the total amount of sugar stored in the body. In other words, it is similar to the total amount stored in a food reservoir. FBS represents the peak value of sugar present in the blood, which was stored in fat cells distributed throughout the body and subsequently released into the blood after depletion of supplied glucose.

Therefore, FBS level drops more slowly than PP2 during the treatment process. It may also increase during prolonged fasting. You should not be surprised as this indicates that a lot of sugar is still stored as fat. FBS begins to drop only when the amount of fat being converted to sugar decreases as a result of regular fasting.

However, once it begins to drop to the normal range, it cascades down like a collapsing sand castle. Therefore, the drop in FBS begins relatively later than PP2 but is a definitive measured value for weight loss and normalization of blood sugar level.

8. **What is glycated hemoglobin and when should it be checked?**

Glycated hemoglobin is expressed as HbA1c or simply A1C. HbA1c represents the number of red blood cells (RBCs) attached to glucose among 100 RBCs[30]. Typically, fewer than 6–7 of 100 RBCs are attached to glucose. However, when blood glucose level increases, the number of RBCs attached to glucose increases. Accordingly, percentage (%) is often used as the unit of HbA1c.

Unlike FBS or PP2, HbA1c can be used to ascertain the average blood sugar level. Since the average value of 2–3 months is often used, checking once every three months, on average, is recommended. Along with FBS, HbA1c is an important observed value. Because it is an averaged value, it does not matter when it is measured, regardless of meals. It is the value with the closest association with diabetes diagnosis, management, and complications[31].

---

[30] The National Institute of Diabetes and Digestive and Kidney Diseases(NIDDK), "Health Information"

[31] Zhang X, Gregg EW, Williamson DF, et al., "A1C level and future risk of diabetes: a systematic review", Diabetes Care, 2010;33(7):1665–1673.

Typically, HbA1c is measured right before or within one week of starting precision diet for diabetes to confirm the peak value. Initially, checking once after two months is recommended. The outcome of precision diet for diabetes tends to be fast; thus, significant decreases are often observed within two months. After sufficiently escaping from diabetes, it is fine to check every three or six months for maintenance and management. HbA1c level is typically measured by testing blood samples at a medical institution or public health center but self-measurement devices similar to self-monitoring glucometers[32] are available that can produce results within five minutes.

[32] Refer to the footnote in "Chapter II-4. For how long should blood sugar levels be checked?"

9.What is the target HbA1c value?

For most adults, the target value for control of type 1 and type 2 diabetes, 7%, is based on significant controversy and discussion about large-scale clinical trials. The unified diagnostic criterion for the diagnosis of diabetes is ≥ 6.5%. There should be no confusion with the diagnostic criterion. Many hypotheses and study results have claimed that lower blood sugar levels could reduce complication and mortality rates. Even today, the absolute majority in the medical community claim as such. However, continuously low blood sugar levels did not prevent complications and adverse events. A prime example is the Action to Control Cardiovascular Risk in Diabetes (ACCORD) study, which reported that excessive lowering of blood sugar level could cause more harm than good. The study was terminated early due to the significantly higher mortality rate in the intensive therapy group (HbA1c 6.4%) compared to that in the standard therapy group (7.5%). The reasons for this unexpected result have not yet been identified.[33]

---

[33] Diabetes Canada Clinical Practice Guidelines Expert Committee, "Diabetes Canada 2018 Clinical Practice Guidelines for the Prevention and Management of Diabetes in Canada", Can J Diabetes, 2018;42(Suppl 1):S1-S325. The section

Recently, a target value of 7% for HbA1c has been proposed in the US; however, the ADA still lists various conditions in which lower values are indicated[34]. Meanwhile, South Korea still uses <6.5% as the control target[35]. Canadian studies and clinical guidelines are recommended since they appear to be most reasonable. The suggested targets are ≤6.5% to lower the risk of chronic renal disease and retinopathy in adults with type 2 diabetes with a low risk of hypoglycemia; ≤7.0% for most adults with type 1 or type 2 diabetes; and 7.1–8.5% for elderly patients who are frail or senile, those with limited life expectancy, and those with repeated hypoglycemic episodes[36].

titled "Targets for Glycemic Control" offers the most comprehensive overview of the controversies regarding DCCT, UKPDS, ACCORD, ADVANCE, VADT, and subsequent studies.

[34] American Diabetes Association, http://www.diabetes.org

[35] Refer to the Korean Diabetes Association, http://www.diabetes.or.kr; The diabetes treatment guidelines amended in June 2019 finally recommends target of 7% for patients with type 1 diabetes and individualized control targets according to patient condition. However, the guidelines still use a target of 6.5% for patients with type 2 diabetes, contrary to international trends.

[36] Refer to Diabetes Canada 2018 Guidelines and website (www.precisiondiabetescare.com) and YouTube channel "Precision Diabetes Care" managed by the author

10. What are the risks and complications of neglected diabetes and the reasons for these conditions?

In the hyperglycemic state, the blood can be described, in somewhat exaggerated manner, as being sticky as highly concentrated sugar water. If hyperglycemia persists, the inner walls of the blood vessels are damaged and the walls thicken during recovery, which causes decreased microvessel flow rates. Consequently, various forms of microvascular complications may appear, which could lead to life-threatening macrovascular complications.

The microvascular complications most requiring monitoring are chronic renal disease and retinopathy. Blockage of retinal microvessels could lead to blurred eyes and poor vision. The kidney does not show specific symptoms until it is completely dysfunctional. Blockage of renal microvessels in the kidney could prevent sufficient blood from the heart through the aorta to enter the renal microvessels, which could cause increased aortic pressure. Consequently, hypertension appears as a symptom. As blockage of renal microvessels worsens over time, the glomerular filtration rate (GFR), the volume of blood filtered per minute by the kidney, significantly decreases. Blood values of blood urea nitrogen (BUN) and creatinine are also important to monitor. This series of processes in which the overall kidney function is lost with increasing microvascular pressure and capillary blockage ultimately leads to chronic renal failure (CRF) in which kidney ceases to function. Then, the only remaining options are dialysis and kidney transplantation. Other microvascular complications include numbness or cold sensation in the hands and feet due to blockage of peripheral blood vessels and Buerger's disease, in which wounds in the tip of the foot do not heal well and fester, leading to toe amputation. Slow healing of skin wounds and itchiness are other common symptoms.

Hypertension occurs from increased aortic pressure due to the blockage of glomerular microvessels in the kidney, resulting in increased cardiac muscle and thickness. At the same time, the inner walls of the blood vessels become clogged and stiffen due to hyperglycemia and hyperlipidemia, which could cause blockage or rupture of macrovessels in the brain and heart. Ultimately, this situation is linked to life and death.

With hyperglycemia, progression into micro- and macrovascular complications is inevitable. A serious problem is that there are almost no perceivable symptoms in the microvascular complication stage. This is the reason why many people are lazy about diabetes care. While people may feel regret once worsening of microvascular complications lead to renal failure or Buerger's disease, worsening of macrovascular complications may not afford the luxury of regret.

Besides direct complications involving micro- and macrovessels in hyperglycemia, hormonal complications are also serious. The levels of insulin secreted in response to soaring blood sugar levels also increase significantly. Fat cells on the liver surface and throughout the body endlessly grow or increase to accelerate fatty liver and obesity. Fat cells on the liver surface are broken down into fatty acid and glycerol and hepatitis may occur due to the destruction of liver cells by fatty acid. If this situation persists, the pancreas may no longer properly secrete insulin. Pancreatic failure and pancreatic cancer have been reported.

Along with the influence at the organ level, increased insulin levels in response to hyperglycemia secondarily inhibits other hormones throughout the body, leading to continued feelings of hunger despite a full stomach by inhibiting secretion of leptin from fat; hypothyroidism; interference with recovery from inflammation by inhibiting secretion of cortisol by the adrenal glands; and infertility, hyposexuality, and polycystic ovarian syndrome by inhibiting male and female sex hormones. The complications caused by the inhibition of hormones can sometimes be handled separately from diabetes; however, one should be aware that they are closely linked. That way, the source of the problem is known and the applicable range of precision diet for diabetes can be determined.

11. Once started, can complications be reversed?

Retinal and renal diseases are important microvascular complications that require monitoring. In most cases, recovery from microvascular complications is possible as long as the hyperglycemic state is well managed. However, once creatinine levels exceed 3 mg/dL[37] due to the progression of renal failure, recovery starts to become very difficult. Recovery may be possible before that point. With retinal disease, recovery of damaged tissues may be difficult but effectively managing blood sugar levels could help to mitigate further progression and promote recovery. Other symptoms such as skin itching and delayed recovery from inflammation, often dissipate naturally as blood sugar level is controlled.

The pattern of macrovascular complications may vary significantly depending on how effectively hypertension, an outcome of microvascular complication, is managed. If the blockage of glomerular microvessels in the kidney is not severe, improvement in GFR by controlling blood

---

[37] While it may vary between laboratories, 0.8–1.2 mg/dL is usually considered the normal range.

sugar level could improve blood pressure(BP) and help to prevent or reduce fatal complications involving the brain and heart. If improvement of the kidneys is difficult, the use of appropriate BP medicine to reduce macrovascular pressure in the brain and heart could be the next best option. However, the sequelae of macrovascular complications are often fatal or difficult to reverse.

Hepatitis, pancreatic failure, and complications due to the inhibition of various hormones are generally reversible. While it may take some time, patients can achieve normal recovery. If blood sugar level is tightly regulated by precision diet for diabetes, insulin levels also drop rapidly to the normal range in response. The forces that inhibited hormones become almost powerless. Excessive appetite is normalized quickly and various problems such as hypothyroidism, chronic inflammation, hyposexuality, infertility, and polycystic ovarian syndrome are gradually addressed as various hormones inhibited by excessive insulin are secreted at normal levels.

12. What are some regular tests that should be performed besides blood sugar level, body weight, and HbA1c for preventing and managing complications?

The monitoring and management of blood sugar level (FBS and PP2), HbA1c, and body weight are important in diabetes[38] to prevent and track complications. Therefore, the physiopathological mechanisms of elevated blood sugar levels need to be observed and blood tests that indicate the sequential process leading up to complications need to be regularly assessed. Once during the initial examination and once every three months thereafter is recommended.

First, there is the lipid test, which measures total cholesterol, TG, HDL, and LDL levels.

A liver function test (LFT) is also needed; namely levels of aspartate aminotransferase (AST or GOT), alanine aminotransferase (ALT or GPT), and gamma(γ)-glutamyl transferase (GGT). Over time, excessive glucose intake

---

[38] Refer to previous items for detailed explanation on this.

causes breakdown of fat stored on the liver surface, which is the primary reservoir, subsequently causing nonalcoholic fatty liver disease (NAFLD) in many cases[39]. It is also important to monitor the degree of liver damage in diabetic patients.

Lastly, monitoring of BUN and creatinine levels and GFR are essential for determining the degree of renal damage.

In addition, annual fundus examination is recommended to check the condition of the retina.

---

[39] A. DP, W.L. P, D.A. C, et al., "Metabolic and nutritional profile of obese adolescents with nonalcoholic fatty liver disease", J Pediatr Gastroenterol Nutr. 2007;44(4):446-452.

III.   Treatment of diabetes

1. What treatment modalities are used in modern medicine?

The reality is that drug therapy[40] is the main option. South Korea, the US, Canada, and England have different criteria and points of emphasis for clinical practice guidelines to address the characteristics and circumstances of patients in their respective countries. According to the 2018 Canadian Clinical Practice Guidelines, which are updated based on the latest research findings, healthy behavioral interventions such as nutritional therapy, weight control, and physical activities are initiated when type 2 diabetes is diagnosed for the first time. In people with HbA1c levels no more than +1.4% above their target (given the target HbA1c level of 7% for most adults with type 1 or type 2 diabetes, this means a range of 7.1–8.4%), drug therapy using metformin is initiated if the target level cannot be reached following three months of healthy behavioral

---

[40] Refer to the following article for the latest details on drug therapy. Cavaiola TS, Pettus JH, "Management of type 2 diabetes: selecting amongst available pharmacological agents. [Updated 2017 Mar 31]", In: Feingold KR, Anawalt B, Boyce A, et al., editors. Endotext [Internet]. South Dartmouth (MA): MDText.com, Inc.; 2000-. Available from: https://www.ncbi.nlm.nih.gov/books/NBK425702/

interventions. When the HbA1c level is higher by at least 1.5% (7.0% + ≥1.5% corresponds to HbA1c ≥8.5%), the combination of healthy behavioral interventions and drug therapy with metformin is used from the start[41], while additional drugs are also considered. Occasionally, insulin may be used from the start in cases involving severe hyperglycemic symptoms or extreme circumstances[42] due to acute diabetes. Additional oral hypoglycemic agents or insulin may also be used depending on the situation. In addition, antihypertensive drugs, antihyperlipidemic drugs, and/or aspirin[43] may be used to prevent complications including cardiovascular disease. In most cases, additional patient education on nutritional or dietary therapy is

[41] The reality is that in primary care, it is all too common to find patients being prescribed and using metformin already for HbA1c exceeding just 6.0%.

[42] They refer to dehydration, diabetic ketoacidosis (DKA), hyperosmolar hyperglycemic syndrome (HHS), etc.

[43] New guidelines from the American Heart Association (AHA), based on a study that reported that the prophylactic use of daily low-dose aspirin offered no benefit to those who without cardiovascular disease or stroke published in March 2019. However, aspirin is still used indiscriminately. Refer to Arnett DK, Blumenthal RS, Albert MA, Buroker AB, Goldberger ZD, Hahn EJ, Himmelfarb CD, Khera A, Lloyd-Jones D, McEvoy JW, Michos ED, Miedema MD, Munoz D, Smith SC Jr, Virani SS, Williams KA Sr, Yeboah J, Ziaeian B., "2019 ACC/AHA guideline on the primary prevention of cardiovascular disease: a report of the American College of Cardiology/American Heart Association Task Force on Clinical Practice Guidelines", Circulation, 2019

conducted in diabetes classes or by clinical nutritionists affiliated with large hospitals.

2. What about drugs for prediabetes or prophylactic purpose?

You are not injured before a traffic accident. Someone who experiences a dangerous situation right before a traffic accident but avoids the accident is not hospitalized for treatment. Because everyone is exposed to the risk of an accident, it is certainly necessary to be careful when walking or driving to avoid a traffic accident on busy roads.

Thus, for individuals with a prediabetic state (FBS of 100–125 mg/dL), it is good to actively emphasize meals, exercise, and weight control. Opinions among physician vary, from the claim that drug prescription is needed in advance to recommending food restriction and exercise without emphasizing anything else, as they would for normal individuals[44]. I support the latter. It is akin to someone taking analgesics for pain that may occur even though he or she did not experience an accident. Remember that prediabetes is not diabetes.

[44] Refer to "Chapter II-2. What is prediabetes?", *The New York Times* article titled "You're 'Prediabetic'? Join the Club", Dec.16, 2016, and commentary on this article in Dr. Younkuk Choi's ECM Eyes, Current Medical News Commentaries

3. Which is better, drug administration or insulin injection? What are the adverse effects of each?

Various types of oral antihyperglycemic drugs all have adverse effects caused by the drug action. While each drug may have different adverse effects, they commonly cause gastrointestinal problems. These drugs lower the concentration of glucose in blood vessels by whatever means; as a result, the amount of glucose sent to the muscles and brain is also reduced. Consequently, the person can easily feel fatigued or lethargic. In severe cases, the person may shake, feel dizzy, or even fall due to the onset of hypoglycemia.

The role of insulin in storing excess glucose in the blood as fat is also linked to the adverse effect of weight gain. In particular, it can cause serious complications[45] by inhibiting other hormones in patients with type 2 diabetes.

Therefore, both antihyperglycemic drugs and insulin require precise prescription and monitoring by the primary physician.

---

[45] Refer to "Chapter II-10. What are the risks and complications of neglected diabetes and the reasons for these conditions?"

The use of insulin is unavoidable for patients with type 1 diabetes. As an alternative, an ongoing study[46] is evaluating insulin placed inside a capsule with a fine needle for absorption by the gastric wall; however, regulation by injection or insulin pump is the current universal method. The amount of insulin use could be reduced significantly by precision diabetes care.

The situation is different for type 2 diabetes. It is certainly manageable without drugs. In fact, drug administration interferes with the escape from diabetes. In rare cases, minimal drugs need to be maintained; however, the number of such cases is very low. It may be beneficial to completely discontinue drugs from the start. In most cases, blood sugar levels drop to the normal range within days to weeks after starting precision diabetes care[47]; however, if the drug is taken out of anxiety, then that could become a relatively excessive dose. As a result, the patient may experience hypoglycemic symptoms; thus, drug

[46] Massachusetts Institute of Technology. "New pill can deliver insulin through the stomach." Science Daily. Feb. 7, 2019.

[47] It is common that the level drops to the normal range on the first day on which the guidelines are accurately learned and practiced. This is not an exaggeration. You can experience and check for yourself.

administration needs to be aggressively reduced or discontinued while monitoring blood sugar levels. Patients who have had type 2 diabetes for decades or more or those who have been taking drugs containing sulfonylurea may experience very slow pancreas recovery and escape from diabetes. In these cases, it may be more beneficial for patients to use and gradually reduce the use of drugs such as metformin.

4. Is it better to keep HbA1c levels lower with drugs and insulin?

Whether by use of oral antihyperglycemic drugs or insulin, lowering HbA1c with drug alone is not effective. Whatever the method, if it is not combined with restricted diet, HbA1c level may not be lowered as expected. In contrast, lowering HbA1c by diet, exercise, and weight control without the use of drugs may be much more effective. You should not make the mistake of thinking that HbA1c level can be managed and long-term complications prevented simply by using a drug or insulin even though you eat as much as you want and do not exercise.

Another major problem is the adverse effect of the long-term use of drugs to artificially lower HbA1c level. The large-scale ACCORD trial reported a significantly increased mortality rate in the intensive control group that achieved an HbA1c level of 6.4%. The results from this study had a definitive impact on adjusting the target HbA1c level to 7% worldwide. In addition, that the results of other large-scale clinical trials such as ADVANCE (Action in Diabetes and Vascular Disease—Preterax and

Diamicron Modified Release Controlled Evaluation) and VADT (the Veterans Affairs Diabetes Trial) observed no significant decrease in the incidence of cardiovascular disease or mortality rate in patients in which HbA1c level was aggressively lowered[48].

[48] Refer to the following article from the American Diabetes Association, which has analyzed and summarized the implications of historic clinical trials including UDDT, UKPDS, ACCORD, ADVANCE, and VADT for observation of favorable and unfavorable outcomes of lower HbA1c levels. Skyler JS, Bergenstal R, Bonow RO, et al. "Intensive glycemic control and the prevention of cardiovascular events: Implications of the ACCORD, ADVANCE, and VA diabetes trials", Diabetes Care, 2009;32(1):187-192.

5. If I have diabetes, must I also take drugs for high cholesterol and hypertension?

Drugs should only be taken when there is a reason to do so. Excessive introduction of glucose into the body due to overeating causes the blood sugar level to increase above the normal level. Surplus glucose also causes TG and LDL levels to increase. Increased blood sugar levels causes thickening of the inner walls of blood vessels from repeated damage and repair. This affects the microvessels distributed through the kidney and retina first and subsequently causes hypertension due to increased pressure in macrovessels. In this situation, lowering the elevated cholesterol level and capillary pressure by reducing the amount of glucose introduced into the body by overeating could result in all problems sequentially returning to normal.

Not addressing overeating that is the cause of these problems and instead forcibly lowering cholesterol level and BP could cause adverse effects for the combined use of these drugs, rather than providing any benefits. Therefore, when precision diabetes care is implemented for type 2 diabetes, there is almost no reason to use drugs for cholesterol or hypertension.

However, there are exceptions. A different approach is needed in cases where escape from diabetes is expected to take a long time due to the long-term use of drugs containing sulfonylurea or decades-long use of a combination of drugs and insulin. It takes time to transition to a situation in which recovery of the pancreas allows glycemic control. In cases with excessively elevated levels in the intermediate process, temporary use of drugs to control cholesterol and BP may offer more advantages than disadvantages. However, this use ultimately becomes unnecessary in most cases. Individuals who are sensitive to the adverse effects of each drug should consult their primary physicians and be even more cautious on their own.

6. Can the treatment modalities used in modern medicine effectively prevent complications?

Historic large-scale clinical trials have shown significant results with respect to the prevention of microvascular complications such as retinopathy, nephropathy, and neuropathy in the intensive control group administered insulin and drugs. However, the role of drug (medicine) in preventing macrovascular complications, including cerebro- and cardiovascular disease (CVD) such as stroke, remains unclear. In the ACCORD trial the preventive effect on CVD was not clear and a significant increase in mortality rate was observed[49].

In conclusion, treatment modalities in modern medicine based mostly on drug administration could play a role in preventing microvascular complications to some degree; however, they may be problematic and limited in preventing macrovascular complications that are directly linked to life and death.

---

[49] Skyler JS, Bergenstal R, Bonow RO, et al., "Intensive glycemic control and the prevention of cardiovascular events: Implications of the ACCORD, ADVANCE, and VA diabetes trials", Diabetes Care, 2009;32(1):187-192.

7. If the treatment modalities used in modern medicine have limitations, then what are the alternatives?

Studies and groups of clinical physicians and researchers recognize the limitations and adverse effects of drug therapy for metabolic disorders, including diabetes, and are active seeking new paths for dietary therapy, defined as the method of eating and types of food eaten. While the numbers of medical professionals and researchers seeking alternatives to diabetes treatment through dietary therapy are still few in numbers, rapid progress is being made since there are definitive and practical effects.

The concept of glycemic index (GI) invented by Dr. David Jenkins[50] from the University of Toronto in Canada is the foundation of the principle for identifying methods to treat diabetes with diet. Subsequently, it has been used widely worldwide based on research led by Jennie Brand-Miller from the University of Sydney in Australia[51]. GI is

[50] Professor of Nutritional Science and Medicine at the University of Toronto after graduating from the University of Oxford in England. He is also a member scientist at the Li Ka Shing Knowledge Institute in St. Michael's Hospital. The concept of glycemic index invented by Dr. Jenkins has been an important basis for attempts to treat diabetes and metabolic disorders by dietary therapy.

expressed as a numeric value between 0 and 100 to indicate how much a specific food increases the blood sugar level in the body. Accordingly, various methods to eat foods with lower GI have been suggested.

Professor Valter Longo from the University of Southern California in the US conducted a study on the cell regeneration effect of FMD and fasting diet[52] that provided basic knowledge on the treatment of diabetes and metabolic disorders. This experimental study is currently in clinical trial[53].

The efforts of Drs. Sarah Hallberg (USA), Jason Fung (Canada), and Andreas Eenfeldt (Sweden) who share the common denominator of low-carb, high-fat, and intermittent fasting (LHIF) are also noteworthy. Dr. Hallberg established an online patient care system based on a low-carb, high-fat diet, has constructed an online patient

---

[51] Boden Institute of Obesity, Nutrition, Exercise and Eating Disorders and Charles Perkins Centre at the University of Sydney; glycemicindex.com

[52] Cheng, Chia-Wel et al., "Fasting-mimicking diet promotes Ngn3-driven β-cell regeneration to reverse diabetes", Cell, 2017

[53] Refer to *The Longevity Diet* by Valter Longo published in January 2018. A Korean version is not available at this time.

management system based on this diet, has joined forces with Virta Health, and is actively pursuing research and business by compiling clinical treatment outcomes[54]. Dr. Fung has been spreading the word about the theoretical mechanisms behind LHIF through his best-selling books *The Obesity Code* and *The Diabetes Code*. He also developed an evidence-based intensive dietary management (IDM) program[55] and is actively engaging in clinical practice and lectures. Dr. Eenfeldt is actively engaged in promotional activities around Sweden to provide theoretical explanations of the therapeutic effects of LHIF for diabetes and metabolic disorders, clinical data collection and introduction, and the development of recipes for practice[56].

Dr. William Li (USA) is known for food research related to cancer prevention and treatment[57] but has more recently described the treatment of diabetes.

---

[54] http://www.virtahealth.com

[55] http://www.idmprogram.com

[56] http://www.dietdoctor.com

[57] If interested, refer to his TED lecture, "Can We Eat to Starve Cancer?" and recent book, *Eat to Beat Disease*

In addition, medical professionals worldwide are changing their perceptions that food, not drugs, is an important therapeutic tool for diabetes and metabolic disorders and are actively sharing their research findings.

In modern medicine, drug therapy remains the predominant modality for diabetes treatment. However, based on the recognition of such limitations, such as in ACCORD, active efforts are underway to identify new way to treat diabetes by diet alone.

8. Could diabetes be completely cured by dietary therapy alone? If so, are there enough international case reports and studies?

Diabetes, especially type 2 diabetes, can be completely cured by dietary therapy alone. The two main issues are what to eat and how to eat. Various methods that have not yet been unified exist, some of which are controversial. However, most methods involve changing what to eat and how to eat, with continued publication of case reports[58] and reliable evidence and study reports[59] on drastic improvement, remission, and maintenance of indicators of diabetes and metabolic disorders such as HbA1c in patients with long histories of type 2 diabetes who have significantly reduced or discontinued their use of drugs and/or insulin.

---

[58] Furmli S, Elmasry R, Ramos M, Fung J., "Therapeutic use of intermittent fasting for people with type 2 diabetes as an alternative to insulin", BMJ Case Rep., 2018:bcr-2017-221854.

[59] McKenzie AL, Hallberg SJ, Creighton BC, Volk BM, Link TM, Abner MK, Glon RM, McCarter JP, Volek JS, Phinney SD, "A novel intervention including individualized nutritional recommendations reduces hemoglobin A1c level, medication use, and weight in type 2 diabetes", JMIR Diabetes, 2017;2(1):e5

The large-scale Diabetes Remission Clinical Trial (DiRECT) in England study investigated the contribution of weight loss through restricted diet on remission of type 2 diabetes. In the first year, the study reported that approximately half of the participants achieved remission to a non-diabetic state even after discontinuing drug administration[60]. The results from the second year were published in the spring of 2019, in which over two-thirds of patients with type 2 diabetes maintained remission, which was associated with the degree weight loss maintenance[61].

Evidence continues to emerge that including dietary therapy in the treatment regimen can help reduce the amount of insulin used in type 1 diabetes cases and that dietary therapy alone could be used to achieve complete remission in type 2 diabetes cases.

---

[60] Lean ME, Leslie WS, Barnes AC, et al., "Primary care-led weight management for remission of type 2 diabetes (DiRECT): an open-label, cluster-randomised trial", Lancet, 2018;391(10120):541-551.

[61] Lean MEJ, Leslie WS, Barnes AC, et al., "Durability of a primary care-led weight-management intervention for remission of type 2 diabetes: 2-year results of the DiRECT open-label, cluster-randomised trial", Lancet Diabetes Endocrinol, 2019;7(5):344-355.

Moreover, the effects are not transient: as long as body weight is well managed after remission, the remission can be sustained.

9. What are the reasons and scientific evidence to support the treatment of diabetes by dietary therapy alone?

The cause of diabetes is often defined as a lack of insulin secretion or the secretion of non-functional insulin due to various lifestyle, genetic, and hormonal problems[62]. The lifestyle problems in type 2 diabetes, which accounts for most cases, include obesity and overweight. Although

---

[62] The National Institute of Diabetes and Digestive and Kidney Diseases (NIDDK), "Health Information Center", https://www.niddk.nih.gov/health-information

[63] Since each individual have a different base rate at which calories are consumed in the body, I do not support the calorie theory. For a simple comparison and understanding, let us assume that you consumed an additional 500 calories and that you are going to exercise to burn the additional calories. To burn those calories, you must run approximately 6 km, which corresponds to approximately 2 hours of walking and 3 hours of hiking. Shawn M. Talbott defined weight control as 75% diet and 25% exercise based on his experience. Based on my own experience, however, weight control is over 90% diet and less than 10% exercise. Refer to "Exercise Vs. Diet: The Truth About Weight Loss" Huffpost, Apr. 30, 2014 (updated Dec. 06, 2017).

While many studies support this opinion, the words and study by Dr. Kelvin Hall from the National Institute of Diabetes and Digestive and Kidney Diseases (NIDDK) at the US National Institute of Health (NIH) are introduced. "If you do go to the gym and you burn all these calories, it takes you so long time to do so and you put in a great amount of effort, you can erase all of that in five minutes of eating a slice of pizza."

Refer to the well-organized article, "Why you shouldn't exercise to lose weight, explained with 60+ studies" Vox, Oct. 31, 2017 and included YouTube video

genetic factors and family history have also been identified, additional research is needed on this topic.

The most common and clear-cut cause of diabetes in most patients are obesity and overweight; ultimately, overeating the main culprit behind these factors. While a lack of exercise and limited physical activity also have influences, they are not definitive. Focusing only on exercise without any diet restrictions is a an ineffective method of weight control[63].

Therefore, more effective weight loss is possible by applying scientific evidence regarding how to eat, such as small portions or regular fasting, and what to eat such as meals with mostly foods with low GI and lowering the percentage of foods with high GI that quickly converted to energy even if the same amount is consumed. This method is directly linked to normalizing type 2 diabetes and achieving remission. The application of the same method to type 1 diabetes could significantly reduce the amount and frequency of insulin use.

10. **What is the best method among immediate transition from drug to dietary therapy, dietary therapy after combination therapy, and continued combination therapy? What is best professional advice to reduce the amount of drug taken?**

The effects of dietary therapy tend to appear immediately in cases involving type 2 diabetes. Therefore, as long as HbA1c level is not $\geq 10\%$, drug therapy could be discontinued and dietary therapy initiated right away. Needless to say, dietary therapy should be administered under the guidance of a specialist well-trained in this field. There are many cases in which the immediate effects of dietary therapy are doubted and the existing drug dose becomes relatively excessive, whereby the adverse effects of hypoglycemia are experienced. During the initial stage of dietary therapy or when using combination therapy with drug therapy for a set period, blood sugar levels should be self-monitored daily to identify trends in blood sugar levels to proactively reduce drug use.

If the HbA1c level is ≥10% at the start, combination therapy with drug therapy may be advisable. However, it is necessary to first eliminate drugs containing sulfonylurea. If used together with insulin injection, it may be beneficial to first discontinue oral antihyperglycemic drug use. Subsequently, the units of insulin could be reduced to eventually discontinue all drug therapy. In rare cases (1 out of 10), combination therapy with drug therapy may be beneficial; thus, the decisions and instructions provided by the specialist should be followed.

11. Are fasting and FMD beneficial for treating diabetes?

Fasting or FMD are essential for treating type 2 diabetes. They may be considered the only methods to calm and reverse insulin and blood sugar levels elevated by overeating. However, irregular fasting must be avoided and only periodic fasting (PF) is acceptable. Even in cases involving type 1 diabetes, fasting or FMD could contribute to the regeneration of pancreatic cells or drastically reduce drug use.

Regularly fasting one or two meals a day, one whole day during the week, and several days during the month are all sound methods. In various cultures, PF is commonly practiced for religious and cultural reasons. Fasting in short cycles could not only help overcome or treat diabetes, obesity, and metabolic disorders but may also offer other health benefits.

There is also sufficient scientific evidence. Professor Valter Longo from the University of Southern California, who published *The Longevity Diet* in January 2018, recommended fasting three to four times a year, about five days each time, based on his own experiments and observations. He proposed that this can maximize the effects of fasting. While there is experimental and clinical evidence and the effects are large, fasting also requires willpower. Dr. Yoshinori Ohsumi of Japan, the 2016 Nobel laureate in physiology or medicine, identified autophagy of damaged cells or toxins during fasting or FMD. If damaged cells or toxins accumulate without such cleaning action by cells, then it becomes difficult to overcome cancer or infectious diseases. Dr. Jason Fung, who is gaining worldwide renown for his application of intermittent fasting (IF) to diabetes and obesity, also advocates the effects of fasting and low-carb diet to his colleagues and patients. Physicians throughout the world have already reported the effects of low-carb and intermittent fasting (LCIF) on diabetes reversal, polycystic ovarian syndrome, infertility, autoimmune disease, and mental and psychological disorders[64].

---

[64] Podcasts such as Dietdoctor or Low Carb MD that began in the second half of 2018 have become venues for sharing opinions and active experiences among experts and physicians in relevant fields.

Fasting is still recommended on a limited basis in the mainstream medical community. However, since physicians and patients worldwide are actively participating in efforts to strengthen its evidence, fasting may soon become the primary treatment modality for escaping from diabetes.

12.   Low-carb, high-fat diet, and ketogenic diets and intermittent fasting have become popular, but are they helpful in treating diabetes?

Numerous dieting methods have been described, including Atkins, Dukan, paleo, and ketogenic diets and IF. In addition, other diets with various methods and goals such as plant-based, vegan, pescatarian, carnivore, low-fat, low-calorie, and Mediterranean diet, have their own evidence and histories. They all exist to achieve weight loss as well as other health and esthetic goals.

Food and diet have always played an ancillary role in treating diseases. The fields in which they are recognized as a central treatment method, similar to drug therapy or surgery, are very few and have very short history. However, as a method for preventing or treating metabolic disorders resulting from overeating, overweight, obesity, diabetes, microvascular complications, macrovascular complications, and ultimately to mortality, it is no longer appropriate that they remain in an ancillary role. Enough scientific validity and medical evidence have been accumulated. At the least, there is sufficient evidence to show that it is unreasonable to continue to use drug therapy as the primary treatment modality. Low-carb diets and/or fasting (including FMD) are just   starting to be applied in medically advanced countries[65]. Alternatives are being identified and realized in places with the capacity to conduct research after using and recognizing the limitations of drug therapy and surgeries as the primary treatment modalities[66].

The popular diets can be divided largely into two types; namely what to eat and how to eat. No matter the name what to eat comes down to the common denominator of the combination of foods with low GI[67]. Moreover, how to eat has the common goal of eating small amount. In other words, the key is the benefit obtained by restricting the

---

[65] Groups of medical professionals In England, Canada, and Australia have formed in recent years to revise national food guides that currently recommend high-carb, low-fat diets. The Public Health Collaboration (England) and Canadian Clinicians for Therapeutic Nutrition (Canada) are prime examples. The government of Western Australia has made aggressive actions since adopting a report stating that low-carb diets are important for the management and remission of patients with type 2 diabetes. Individual physicians and research groups are highly active in the US, whereas recognition by the medical community remains weak in South Korea. Refer to "Landmark diabetes report says low-carb is a top option" Diet Doctor, Apr. 19, 2019. http://www.dietdoctor.com

[66] Refer to "Section III-7. If the treatment modalities used in modern medicine have limitations, then what are the alternatives?"

[67] The research groups led by Dr. David Jenkins from the University of Toronto in Canada and Jennie Brand-Miller from the University of Sydney in Australia, as explained in Section III-7, have made profound basic scientific contributions.

total amount of food intake by soothing, fooling, or even ignoring one's appetite.

Therefore, while the advantages, disadvantages, and efficiency differ with respect to treating diabetes, no matter the method or name is, as long as the dietary therapy inherently adheres to the two principles of foods with low GI and eating less, it can not only help the escape from diabetes but could also be the most important treatment choice.

13. What is the best dietary therapy?

The transition from drug to dietary therapy as the most important method for the treatment of diabetes is progressing with increasing evidence[68]. It may be confusing at times to determine which is the best among various dietary therapy methods that have been introduced.

Check to see if the following four conditions are satisfied. Firstly, does the diet mostly recommend foods with low GI? Typically, rice or bread (and most grains) have GI values close to the maximum of 100. Accordingly, many dietary therapies recommend low-carb diets. Proteins from fish and meat do not contain carbohydrates; thus, they are excluded from measurement. Proteins typically play a role in creating human tissues rather than being used directly as energy. However, estimation and comparison of the degrees of energy supply by different pathways and contexts shows that protein also plays a role in the gradual supply of moderate amounts of energy. Vegetables except for root vegetables generally have low GI ; thus, caution is

---

[68] Refer to "Chapter III-8 Could diabetes be completely cured by dietary therapy alone? If so, are there enough international case reports and studies?" for further information.

needed regarding the amount of root vegetables consumed. Intake of high-GI foods must be reduced. Secondly, what is the total meal size? The amount of food must not exceed the total daily energy requirements for metabolism and exercise. Based on the activity level required for regular office work, most modern people tend to eat too much. While it is difficult to generalize, it is necessary to check whether you are eating because you are hungry or eating habitually because it is time to eat even though you are not hungry. Moreover, you should also check if you are eating until you become full or eating to the point of feeling not quite full. Thirdly, does the diet recommend regular meals? Fourthly, does it recommend an individualized precision diet?

If all of the four conditions are satisfied, then it could be the best dietary therapy. Dietary therapies with primary goals of reversing diabetes could offer additional benefits in disease prevention and esthetic and psychological improvement through weight loss. Diets satisfying the first and second conditions have started to receive recognition for their value since studies and clinical trials conducted worldwide have reported their positive effects on diabetes and weight control. There is no "best" diet that satisfies the third and fourth conditions. That is the reason for the introduction of precision diabetes care (PDC) based on precision diets for diabetes.

IV.   Precision diet for diabetes

1. What is the precision diet for diabetes and what specific methods does it involve?

The term "precision" is the latest version of the terms "personalized" and "individualized"[69]. Various dietary therapy methods exist to treat diabetes. Their common points are low carbohydrates and fasting or FMD. The method is worthwhile. Moreover, there is sufficient scientific and medical evidence of its effectiveness. Although it is still considered a minority opinion, it is becoming more well known through the increasing number of physicians, researchers, and experiencers worldwide[70]. This is welcome news. However, it also has a critical problem. Precision diet for diabetes is the near-perfect

---

[69] The term was borrowed from Precision Medicine. The definition given by the US NIH Precision Medicine Initiative is "an emerging approach for disease treatment and prevention that takes into account individual variability in genes, environment, and lifestyle for each person." It is being used interchangeably as an upgraded term for personalized, individualized, and customized. This may be most similar to the concept of "constitution" that has long been applied in Traditional Korean Medicine for disease prevention and treatment. As will be explained further, the most important basis of the diabetes treatment method designed by the author is the application of a dietary therapy with diets that vary in type and method for each individual; therefore, the concept of "precision" is applied appropriately and "precision diabetes care" was newly created accordingly.

[70] Refer to "Chapter III: Treatment of diabetes"

dietary therapy that I designed to address this problem on the basis of my research and experience as a physician at the frontline treating diabetes and metabolic disorders[71]. The core principle is that meal types and methods must vary for each individual. That is the reason why the term "precision" was added. As a method that has been applied in primary care for nearly two decades and passed on to many fellow physicians to achieve similar revolutionary outcomes of curing type 2 diabetes, its efficacy has been clinically proven. An ongoing challenge is to collect and publish cases involving the cure of type 2 diabetes as research data to establish academic evidence.

The method involves four key factors. **The foremost is to practice PF or FMD.** Type 2 diabetes is a series of events involving elevated glucose levels in the body due to overeating,[72] elevated insulin level, and dysfunction nearing pancreatic failure. These are reversible processes

---

[71] It is believed that a "perfect" dietary therapy is the work of God.

[72] Overeating grains with high GI is most problematic but overeating any nutrient, even proteins and fats, causes a buildup of surplus energy, which, in turn, could cause various metabolic disorders, including diabetes. Therefore, diets that advocate eating unrestricted amounts of meat or vegetables, as long as grains are avoided, are often problematic. The intake of minimal amounts of appropriate grains is essential and beneficial.

that can be normalized by reducing food intake to very low levels. Therefore, a complete cure is possible. Using various types of antihyperglycemic agents to suppress the intermediate processes without controlling overeating, the starting point, is only a temporary measure and the reason why a complete cure cannot be achieved with drug therapy alone. In most cases, overeating can be defined as feeling full after a meal. You should remember the golden rule about filling only about 80% of your stomach. You reach that point when you feel that you want to eat just a little bit more. The actual method of FMD is to determine the meal size that would cause you to feel hungry 30 minutes to an hour before your next meal. Other methods include reducing the number of meals per day to two or just one to sufficiently increase the fasting time, regular fasting every other day, one day per week, or a few days per month. In particular, for people with HbA1c levels $\geq 10\%$, fasting for

three days or every other day at the start may be a sound method. You should adopt the habit of enjoying hunger. You should also make an effort to form a habit of eating a restricted diet for the rest of your life and not just for a set period. You should be cautious to practice this method under the supervision and instructions of a relevant specialist. **The second factor is strict control of the proportions of vegetables, meat, and grains to 100:60:(0–)20.** In this way, you not only eat a minimal amount but also strictly restrict the glucose level in your body. Carbohydrates, the main constituents of grains, have the fastest rate of conversion to glucose and, thus, energy. Accordingly, activities and cognitive ability from energy derived from glucose used by the brain and muscles disappear in about one hour and it could have adverse effects in diabetic patients. Drastic increases in glucose levels cause excessive insulin secretion, leading to a vicious cycle of being unable to resist the desire to eat more. While carbohydrates are an essential nutrient that provide rapid power and contribute to metabolism, only a minimal amount should be consumed. For diabetic patients with HbA1c levels <10%, carbohydrates should comprise a maximum of 20% of the meal, corresponding approximately a quarter of the palm in size. For severely diabetic patients with HbA1c levels ≥10%, it may be necessary to maintain 0% carbohydrate consumption for the first few weeks to months. Since the nutrients provided by carbohydrates are stored in large amounts in the body, they do not need to be consumed for a while. Slightly higher proportions of carbohydrates (exceeding 20% or quarter-palm size) is acceptable for individuals with jobs that require significant muscle use, athletes, and highly active children. Protein, the main constituent of meat, is an essential nutrient used to build tissues in the body; it is preferably not used for conversion to energy. When necessary, protein can be partially converted to glucose for use as energy. However, it has a longer gastrointestinal retention time and is converted to glucose only in specific circumstances[73]. Because this conversion takes a relatively long time, it has the effect of continuously maintaining a moderate energy level. At the same time, it does not facilitate insulin secretion. Therefore, it is a relatively safe nutrient for diabetic patients; thus, meals should comprise approximately 60% protein, corresponding to approximately a half-palm size. Fat, which is one of three

---

[73] A part of glyconeogenesis

major nutrients, should be consumed in small amounts by choosing the type that is suitable for you; alternatively, the amount contained in meat should be sufficient. There are not many reasons for consuming high amounts of fat; thus, it does not have a significant presence in the precision diet for diabetes. Vegetables contain small amounts of carbohydrates and are rich in fiber. They tend to have low GI due to their low carbohydrate content; thus, relatively large amounts can be consumed. The recommended proportion is 100%, corresponding to a palm-size measure. Sufficient dietary fiber is helpful for satiety and bowel movements; thus, it is used to compensate for relative deprivation due to FMD. Due to their relatively high GI, the amount of root vegetables consumed must be properly controlled. Although potatoes and sweet potatoes are classified as vegetables, they have high GIs, close to those of grains, and should be consumed at the same percentage as that for grains. **The third factor in the precision diet is regular meals.** Whether one, two, or three meals a day, mealtime(s) must be set consistently depending on your life patterns and diabetes severity. While *"intermittent"* fasting (IF) is available, it should be modified to *"periodic"* fasting (PF). While it may work as a method of FMD, it could be disadvantageous if the regularity of the human body is ignored. Irregular eating, sleeping, waking, and going to the bathroom cause the body to prepare for crises. Irregular eating causes the body to prepare for hunger situations and store everything inside the body, regardless of the size of the meals. In contrast, if you eat regularly but occasionally overeat or not on time, the body does not store nutrients in such an extreme manner. Therefore, irregular meals lead to more storage despite eating less, which leads to the frustration of gaining weight despite eating little and increasing the risk of diabetes, as well as delaying the escape from diabetes. **The fourth factor that should not be overlooked is choosing the types of foods that are right for you.** This is the key among keys in the precision diet for diabetes. People can be divided into types according to meals that they mostly eat; namely, beef and root vegetables (Beef, Type B), pork and mostly vegetables (Pork, Type P), chicken and spicy vegetables (Chicken, Type C), and seafood and leafy vegetables (Seafood, Type S)[74]. Such divisions are based

on diagnoses by specialists[75]. If the types of food are not beneficial to you, you may experience delayed glycemic control or adverse effects such as dermatitis, indigestion, abdominal distention, lethargy, and flu-like symptoms[76]. One option would be to try meals from a specific group for one or two months according to your preferences or reactions and observe the results to find the group that is right for you. Needless to say, professional assistance and advice are of utmost importance.

---

[74] Details about the types of food for each group are provided in Appendix II

[75] There are various claims about how to find foods that are right for you. They can be categorized by genetic testing or comparative analyses based on preferences, tastes, reactions, and medical history. Traditional medicine in each country worldwide has ways of categorizing foods that are beneficial or harmful based on their own theories and evidence. The author determined that Eight Constitution Medicine of Korea was best at researching and analyzing the relationships between human diseases and foods and used it as the basis for categorization.

[76] Keto rash, keto flu, gout, bad breath, constipation, and elevated cholesterol level, which are common adverse effects associated with low-carbohydrate and ketogenic diets, are likely to result from not finding the types of food that are right for you.

2. What are some differences between the precision diet for diabetes and dietary therapy for diabetes taught in diabetes classes at regular hospitals?

According to the latest guidelines followed by each hospital in South Korea, the US, and Canada,[77] dietary therapy is still not at the center of treatment. Their position is that diabetes cannot be treated by lifestyle intervention (including dietary therapy) alone and, when combined with drug therapy, it plays only an assisting role. Recommendations to avoid overeating and to eat grains with low carbohydrate content or fiber-rich vegetables are relatively common. No specific methods are suggested; the guidelines only contain principle-based content about controlling weight by receiving guidance from a professional nutritionist and eating balanced meals by choosing a meal plan that suits each individual. This is

---

[77] Korean Diabetes Association, Treatment Guideline for Diabetes, sixth edition, May 2019.

American Diabetes Association, "5. Lifestyle Management: Standards of Medical Care in Diabetes-2019", Diabetes Care, 2019 Jan; 42(Supplement 1):S46-S60.

Diabetes Canada Clinical Practice Guidelines Expert Committee, "Diabetes Canada 2018 Clinical Practice Guidelines for the Prevention and Management of Diabetes in Canada", Can J Diabetes, 2018;42(Suppl 1):S1-S325.

likely due to the presumption that diabetes cannot be treated by dietary therapy alone. The guidelines place a greater emphasis on the trivial disadvantages of dietary therapy rather than its major advantages that allow a complete cure of type 2 diabetes[78]. They still claim out-of-fashion calorie counting and low-fat diets as proof. The education and instruction provided by regular diabetes classes actually prevent many diabetic patients from breaking free from conventional beliefs and educate people that diabetes is incurable.

The academic evidence of the effects of a lifestyle intervention based on dietary therapy on reducing the use of drugs among patients with type 1 diabetes and completely curing patients with type 2 diabetes has been described thoroughly in the previous chapters of this book. Basically, choosing foods with low GI through FMD and low-carb diet is the common point. Despite this, there are some insufficiencies. There is no perfection in research and development by humans. Precision diet for diabetes

---

[78] US ADA guidelines present the disadvantages in a more detailed and aggressive manner. Refer to previous citation, "5. Lifestyle Management: Standards of Medical Care in Diabetes-2019"

represents some modifications and supplementation to make it closer to perfect, meaning sustaining long-term remission without short-term adverse effects[79]. Specifically, two more factors are added; namely, regular mealtimes and choosing foods according to your personal type. This becomes a sustainable method to completely discontinue drug therapy without adverse effects and escaping from diabetes to guarantee a lifetime of healthy living.

---

[79] This method was discovered, tested, and completed by the author on the basis of his clinical experience in treating diabetic patients for approximately 10 years before various diabetes-curing diets, often referred as low-carb and intermittent fasting (LCIF), became trendy. Because it was not publicized in Korea and English-speaking countries, it may be mistaken as have been developed after LCIF became trendy by simply supplementing some parts that were lacking. Long before such trends, the precision diet for diabetes was established with the four basic pillars of FMD, selection of foods with low GI/GL, regular mealtime, and food choices according to the type of person. The keystone of precision diabetes care is providing real-time care through digital technology by promoting lifestyle changes based on the overall type of each person by adding lifestyle interventions, such as exercise, bathing, and breathing techniques for each type of person, to the precision diet.

3. What are the differences between low-carbohydrate, high-fat, and intermittent fasting and precision diets for diabetes?

The position that diabetes cannot be treated by dietary therapy alone and the opposing position both share two common points; low-carbohydrate diets with low GI and avoiding overeating[80]. There is controversy regarding high-fat diets. The low-carb, high-fat (LCHF) & intermittent fasting (IF) method advocated by Dr. Jason Fung and Dr. Sarah Hallberg has spread throughout the eastern part of North America. Based on the types of foods recommended, the people who succeeded with this diet may have been the types of people for whom meats and fat were suitable. In contrast, the diet advocated by Professor Valter Longo in the western US consisted mostly of vegetables and fish in addition to periodic fasting (PF) on the basis of his ethnic background and experimental and observational studies[81]. Many people achieved good results with this diet and a clinical trial is being conducted. How should we interpret

---

[80] While claims differ regarding methods for fasting mimicking diet and fasting, there is the unified opinion that overeating should be avoided.

[81] Valter Longo, *The Longevity Diet*, 2018

the amazing results achieved with diets that seem to have almost opposite food types?

This is obvious from the perspective of precision diet for diabetes, in which the key is to choose the types of foods with low GI according to the type of person and regularly practicing FMD. Improvement in blood sugar level and body weight but the appearance of adverse effects, such as dermatitis, indigestion, and general weakness from eating meats and foods with high fat content may also be attributed to choosing types of foods that are not suitable for one's own type. In contrast, restoration of a diabetic pancreas without adverse effects from regular FMD consisting mostly of vegetables and fish could only be achieved in people for whom those types of foods are suitable. The additional consumption of fat is not generally recommended in the precision diet for diabetes as the fat contained in fish and meat comprising 60% of the meal is sufficient.

4. What are glycemic index, glycemic load, and insulin index?

Accurate quantification of the rate and magnitude of blood sugar increases when certain foods and the effects on insulin secretion then such values could be useful in differentiating and controlling the types of food eaten. These measures include GI[82] and GL[83]. Recently, the use has expanded to include the insulin index[84].

---

[82] D J Jenkins, T M Wolever, R H Taylor, H Barker, H Fielden, J M Baldwin, A C Bowling, H C Newman, A L Jenkins, D V Goff, "Glycemic index of foods: a physiological basis for carbohydrate exchange", Am J Clin Nutr, 34(3);1981:362-366.

The concept of glycemic index was first introduced in this article and ignited a heated debate. In the article, the glycemic index for ice cream and bread is much lower than that for rice. For details about this controversy, refer to the article by Phil Tucker, titled "How the Glycemic Index Lies to You." Without being aware of this article, the author compared weights on the days after eating rice versus ice cream and found that weight increased less after eating ice cream. After this experience, the existence of the glycemic index was realized.

[83] After the initial publication of the study on GI by Dr. David Jenkins at the University of Toronto in Canada, the University of Sydney in Australia conducted studies on the GI of individual foods. These values can be searched in http://www.glycemicindex.com. The Glycemic Index Foundation, affiliated with the same university, is currently conducting studies on GL and insulin index. Refer to https://www.gisymbol.com.

[84] The insulin index is searchable on the homepage of Nutrita, a company founded by Portuguese scientist Raphael Sirtoli.

In GI, the rate at which pure glucose is absorbed by blood vessels is set at 100 so that the rates at which certain foods are digested and converted into blood glucose can be compared and expressed as numeric values. Although it has the limitation of significant variation depending on the cooking method, degree of ripeness, combination with other components, and individual differences in metabolism, GI still provides basic information that could be used when choosing food. Values ≤ 55, 56–69, and ≥ 70 are considered low, moderate, and high GI, respectively. GI represents the rates at which carbohydrates are broken down and converted to glucose. Because fat and meat proteins cannot be measured for GI, their assigned value is 0. Proteins and fat slow digestion; thus, they also play an indirect role in lowering GI by slightly delaying the conversion of carbohydrates.

Although GI reflects the degree of influence that a specific food has on blood sugar level, GI varies according to how much of that food is consumed. In other words, consideration must be given to when food with a high GI is consumed in small amounts versus when food with a low

GI is consumed in large amounts. As an example, let us assume you ate 120 g of watermelon. Experimental results showed a high GI of 80. Much of that 120 g comprised water and fibers; thus, carbohydrates accounted for 6 g. The formula for calculating GL is GI x carbohydrate mass (g) divided by 100; in this case, (80 x 6 g)/100 = 4.8 or approximately 5. GL values ≤ 10, 11–19, and ≥ 20 are considered low, moderate, and high, respectively. Accordingly, the example given above has a high GI of 80, but a very low GL of 5. Thus, people with diabetes or metabolic disorder can eat watermelon with little concern for increased blood sugar levels. As shown, GL is a better indicator and GI to estimate the actual influence of a food on blood sugar level. Therefore, wisdom should be exercised to choose foods with low GL among foods that are suitable for you.

	Glycemic Index (GI)	Glycemic Load (GL)
High	70 ↑	20 ↑
Mild	56~69	11~19
Low	55 ↓	10 ↓

For reference, the insulin index is a value reflecting how much insulin is secreted in the body at two hours after consuming a specific food. The level of insulin secretion at two hours after consuming pure glucose is set to the reference value of 100. Each food has a variety of constituents that have complex influences on hormones and metabolism. Since there may be significant differences according to the type of individual, the efficacy of insulin index requires further scrutiny as it is not yet universally accepted.

In conclusion, the current measurements available for relatively close approximations of the influences of certain foods on the body in relation to metabolic disorders including diabetes include GI, amount of carbohydrates in a reference volume, GL is calculated based on those values and insulin index. All foods have different constituents, as well as functional aspects related to how they interact with individual organs and structural differences within the body itself, such as differences in intestinal length, lung size, and other physiological functions.

Therefore, while these values cannot be truly accurate, they can be used for reference.

5. What are the differences between calorie-restricted and glucose-restricted diets?

"Calorie is dead"[85]. The calorie theory, an effort to identify the influence of foods on the human body, deserves to be abandoned and should have been abandoned long ago. The value is fixed at 4-4-9 kcal per 1 g of carbohydrates-protein-fat. Using the analogy of the human body being a coal furnace, burning carbohydrates generates 4 kcal of heat, assuming complete combustion. If coal is wet or there is not enough oxygen, incomplete combustion could occur and not even 1 kcal of heat may be generated. In contrast, additional oxygen may result in the generation of more than 5–6 kcal of heat. It is an overly simplified assumption to claim that 1 g of carbohydrates always generates 4 kcal of heat without accounting for a wide range of variables such as the condition of the material itself, metabolic rate, degree of digestion, and the structure and function of organs inside the human body, which is

---

[85] This is from the article titled "Death of the Calorie" that appeared in the special science edition of the magazine *The Economist 1843*. While many long have pointed out the problem of calorie calculation and advocated its abandonment, the article by Peter Wilson that appeared in the April/May 2019 edition best illustrates the point. You may be able to gain useful knowledge from reading the full text.

obviously more complex than a coal furnace. The number of calories generated could vary significantly according to numerous variables. Therefore, calorie counts based on such simple numeric values are highly inaccurate. Erroneous calorie counts that have been used for over a century are still used in various fields despite counter-arguments. This persistent use is causing significant harm in the field of medicine, leading to recommendations to consume less high-calorie fat. Among the etiologies of heart disease, fat has been blamed as the main culprit for diabetes, hyperlipidemia, and obesity, while guidelines have described fat as something bad that should be reduced to extreme levels due to high calories. However, the real culprit is overeating carbohydrates that are unsuitable for one's self[86].

Efforts to quantify the degree of influence of food on the human body are obviously needed. GI emerged due to the

---

[86] Studies have compared the weight controlling effects between diets with reduction of daily intake of high-calorie fat to below 35% and those with reduction of daily intake of carbohydrates to below 130 g. The Public Health Collaboration formed by British physicians published the results of their comparison of 26 randomized controlled trials (RCTs). All 26 RCTs showed statistically significant results in the low-carb group, whereas no study showed significant results in the low-fat group. Refer to http://phcuk.org/RCTs/ for detailed comparisons.

inaccuracy of counting calories[87]. The GI is a numeric value that reflects the rate at which carbohydrates are converted to glucose and subsequently cause increased blood glucose levels. While the GI is also based on many imperfect variables, its influence on the human body is more realistic than that of calories. GL, which is calculated based on the GI and amount of carbohydrates contained in the food consumed, could supplement what GI may lack in identifying the influence on obesity, diabetes, and metabolic disorders. The insulin index was introduced to analyze how insulin is secreted in the body by reacting sensitively to the influence of glucose introduced into the body, but it has not been universally accepted. This index comes closer to determining the actual influence of certain foods on diabetes, obesity, and metabolic disorders. However, determining how the same food may differently affect an individual requires further assessment[88]. The

---

[87] Refer to the previous chapter

[88] Among various studies, the most well-known is the 2015 study by Israeli researchers that demonstrated individual responses to PP2 for the same food. The differences were attributed to the gut microbiome, which has become a trendy field of research worldwide. However, the author's opinion is that the reason is due to structural differences in the body that cause different distributions of the gut microbiome. Zeevi D, Korem T, Zmora N, et al., "Personalized nutrition by

principle that "Not everybody is the same," as advocated by the precision diet for diabetes, is a difficult problem to solve without prioritizing the basic presuppositions. Specifically, one must start with the fact that there exist differences based on the structure of organs and their relative strengths and weaknesses to identify the clues.

Ongoing research and advances have advanced just enough for use as references; however, these values cannot be accurate unless one first differentiates the various human body responses according to different human types. By simply referencing these, the restriction of foods with high GI and GL, which cause especially high insulin levels in the body, according to the principle of precision diet for diabetes will allow complete long-term escape from diabetes without any adverse effects.

---

prediction of glycemic responses", Cell, 2015;163(5):1079-1094. Also refer to the ongoing Personalized Nutrition Project conducted by the authors of this paper; http://www.personalnutrition.org

6. Does the precision diet for diabetes not consider calorie counts at all?

The precision diet does not consider calories at all. This is because how calories are counted in physics differs from how they are used in the human body and is completely unrelated to their influences on human physiology or diseases[89]. While they may currently have some inaccuracies, the indices that influence human physiology and pathology include GI, GL, and insulin index. Moreover, measuring food weight is more practical than counting calories.

Refer to the table below, which was constructed by the author using personally collected data. Let us compare beef (210 kcal) and white bread (219 kcal), which have similar calories per 100 g. Let us assume that type B or P people, for whom both types of food are beneficial, practice the precision diet for diabetes care or weight control. Even though they consume similar calories, those who continue to eat white bread will not lose weight and may instead

---

[89] Refer to "Chapter IV-5. What are the differences between calorie-restricted and glucose-restricted diets?" and corresponding citations.

gain weight. If they are diabetic, their blood sugar levels will also increase. This is because the GI of white bread, which reflects its rate of conversion to glucose after consumption and digestion, is 71, while its GL is 8–24. Both of these values are very high and even the insulin index, which reflects the degree to which it induces insulin production, is also very high at 58–77%. In contrast, those who consume the same number of calories of beef may lose weight and have a stable blood sugar level. Since GI and GL are used to measure the influence of carbohydrates in the body, fat or protein cannot be measured. However, glucose generated by glyconeogenesis is maintained for a long time below a moderate level. At the same time, the insulin index of beef (27%) is much lower than that of white bread (58–77%). Therefore, beef is a very beneficial food for weight and diabetes control.

	Calories/100g	Glycemic Index	Glycemic Load	Insulin Index
Lettuce	13	15	1	34%
Carrot	41	39-49	2	45%
Fish	80~116	X	x	29%
Beef steak	210	X	x	27%
White bread	219	71	8~24	58~77%
White rice	129	72	16-30	45%

※ GI, GL: glycemicindex.com
Insulin Index: nutrita.app

There have been claims that a calorie-restricted diet can result in weight loss for a certain period and improved blood sugar levels. This is because grams of food, meaning the absolute amount of food, were reduced to limit calories. However, a study that compared low-carbohydrate and calorie-restricted low-fat diets did not observe statistically significant results for any participant[90].

---

[90] Refer to the articles in citation #87.

7. How can I find the types of foods that are right for me?

Many researchers and clinicians agree a "one-drug-fits-all" approach is no longer acceptable in modern medicine. However, opinions vary on how standards should be set. The US NIH, which defined precision medicine, indicated that disease treatment and prevention should consider genetic and environmental factors as well as individual patient lifestyles. Since 2015, the applicable range of this approach has broadened in various fields of western medicine, including chronic diseases and cancer. This is very fortunate and desirable. There remains a tendency to focus only on genes, but diverse reasons, including the gut microbiome, are gradually being identified. Accordingly, studies are collecting food reaction data from individuals and using artificial intelligence to predict the beneficial or harmful effects of specific foods.

With respect to escaping from diabetes, obesity, and metabolic disorders, low carbohydrate consumption and FMD are at least close to the truth based on medical and scientific mechanisms and actual evidence and experiences from clinical trials. The problem is the specific methods. Broadly, the typical methods are carnivore and vegetarian diets. Moreover, many studies have reported how the same foods may show different elevations in blood sugar levels depending on the individual person[91]. If so, how should this be differentiated?

Objective tools for clear differentiation are still lacking. However, we cannot wait until they become available. One option is to test one's reaction[92], but it is not easy. Such attempts should be made under the guidance of a specialist. Erroneous reactions may appear depending on the gastrointestinal tract or health conditions. PP2 should be measured, but it is also necessary to observe and record details related to digestion, voiding status, general fatigue, and skin conditions over several weeks to months. If uncomfortable symptoms appear, the method should be abandoned and another method tried. Among the dietary

[91] Refer to citation #89.

[92] Search for a story about a young woman named Mikhaila Peterson. Her tireless food testing allowed complete escape from autoimmune disease and depression that she had suffered for over 20 years. She only consumed beef, water, and salt. She is actively telling her own story and method on SNS; however, this method is applicable only to her. It is impractical to insist that everyone should be on extreme meat diet.

therapies according to by four types presented in the precision diet for diabetes,[93] one could be selected arbitrarily for testing based on individual preferences and reactions. Of course, diagnosis by a specialist from a relevant field[94] is best for specific typing. Lastly, if you already know what types of food are good for you, by whatever means, then one of type B, P, C, or S could be selected and FMD, regular meals, and proper proportions (vegetable-meat-grain: 100-60-(0)~20) can be practiced immediately. You can not only quickly escape from diabetes but also metabolic disorders and obesity. As a bonus, you will also achieve lifelong healthy living.

---

[93] Refer to Appendix II

[94] Dr. Dowon Kuon of Korea divided humans into eight types and founded Eight Constitution Medicine (ECM), which was introduced internationally in 1965 in Tokyo, Japan. The relationship between human diseases and food was clinically analyzed most precisely and actually applied for use in treating various intractable diseases, including cancer. The author of this book is a physician who specializes in ECM who realized during lengthy clinical practice that diabetes and metabolic disorders belong to a disease group that could be cured by considering food amounts and proportions. The precision diet for diabetes was devised by simplifying Dr. Dowon Kuon's ECM diet to help anyone to easily escape from diabetes. Many physician colleagues have been professionally trained and are practicing method. Refer to http://www.ecmclinic.com.

8. When practicing the precision diet for diabetes, how do I measure the amount of food?

The precision diet for diabetes is based on FMD. The methods for determining the amount of food for FMD that is right for you are as follows. If you eat three meals a day, breakfast should be smaller than normal; you should then determine whether you feel hungry at 30 minutes to an hour before lunch. If you are not hungry, then the amount of breakfast was too much. For lunch, eat only half of the amount eaten for breakfast and again determine whether you are hungry at 30 minutes to an hour before dinner. Feeling hungry is considered light eating. After a few attempts, you should be able to determine your personal meal size for light eating. This is the most important first guidance.

Some people do not feel hungry despite using this method. If they have no digestive disorder[95], then the number of meals per day could be reduced to two or one. Another option is to fast every other day. The key is whether you

---

[95] When someone has a digestive disease, appetite and hunger may not be consistent. In such cases, the method must be altered as instructed by a specialist.

feel hungry enough before a meal. You need to be trained to enjoy hunger.

For patients with very severe hyperglycemia (HbA1c level $\geq 10\%$), fasting for the first 3–5 days[96] may be beneficial.

Care should be taken to check blood sugar levels and aggressively reduce the use of insulin or anti-diabetic drugs. The effects of fasting or FMD are almost immediate; thus, maintaining the same drugs could cause hypoglycemia due to overmedication. Therefore, fasting or FMD should be performed under the guidance of a specialist.

In nature, only humans eat food for fun and not just for fuel. Humans are almost the only organisms to die from diseases, except for livestock fed and raised by humans. In nature, wild animals mostly starve to death, freeze to death, or get eaten by another animal but do not die from diseases as humans do[97]. A quantitative surplus goes beyond obesity

---

[96] Another effective method could be FMD one day and fasting on the following day.

[97] Rare exceptions include the high rates of cancer among elephants in zoos and beluga whales (*Delphinapterus leucas*) that feed on hazardous substances in the ocean. Refer to https://www.ncbi.nlm.nih.gov/pmc/articles/PMC1240769/pdf/ehp0110-000285.pdf

and becomes a direct cause of diabetes and metabolic disorders. Likewise, it is the same for a qualitative surplus of mostly carbohydrates. Like feeding meat to an herbivore like a cow, serious diseases such as chronic inflammation, hormone disruption, and autoimmune disease could be the long-term outcomes of eating foods not suitable for one's self. These habits could also cause of type 1 diabetes or various intractable chronic diseases.

9. What are some ways to overcome hunger during FMD?

In most cases, hyperglycemia causes hyperinsulinemia, while elevated insulin levels may induce perturbances of the feeding center by inhibiting the leptin hormone. This condition further induces binge eating. Insulin injections cause insulin levels inside the body to increase rather than decrease. Therefore, drugs used for diabetes cause even more hunger and ultimately paradoxically exacerbate diabetes.

There is no other method besides drastically reducing the amount of glucose introduced into the body. When implementing the precision diet for diabetes, it may be difficult to withstand hunger for the first several days after starting FMD, which can be attributed to insulin not initially dropping to an appropriate level despite the drastic decrease in glucose intake. In most cases, the level will decrease rapidly and no longer cause excessive appetite but this change may take several days. Occasionally, sharp increases in insulin levels may occur from an inability to resist binge eating.

One method to temporarily fool the feeding center is to slowly sip water when severe hunger is felt. Warm water is recommended for types B and C, while lukewarm or cool water is recommended for types P and S[98]. Water should not be gulped all at once. Finding and drinking tea that is beneficial to you is a good method too. It must be sipped to fool the stomach and brain to escape and resist sudden hunger.

---

[98] Refer to Appendix II.

10. How much weight should people with type 2 diabetes lose?

The fact that escape from type 2 diabetes is possible by losing weight is shown through experience and study results. Most people who are overweight or obese need to lose weight. While there are different opinions about how much weight to lose, studies generally report that losses of 5–10% to be beneficial.

In precision diabetes care (PDC), the weight loss goal is set to about 10% on the basis of lengthy clinical experience and observations. The reference weight is the weight that was consistently maintained for at least 10 years during the healthiest period in life during the patient's 20s or 30s. For example, consider a middle-aged woman who maintained a weight of 50 kg for at least 10 years during her 20s and 30s when she was healthy who currently weighs 70 kg. Her weight goal for escaping diabetes should be 45–55 kg based on ± 10% of 50 kg. That means she needs to lose at least 15 kg. Excessive weight loss of 10% to reach the goal of 45 kg may be unrealistic and cause health problems. Furthermore, you should be very careful about losing 3–4 kg or more a month. A weight loss of approximately 1 kg a week or 3~4 kg a month is the maximum amount of weight that can be lost without health concerns. While it is possible to lose even more weight in this time, the body may not be able to handle the loss. In the example given above, practicing the precision diet for diabetes with a target of losing 15 kg over 4–5 months could allow a healthy escape from diabetes. For the optimal effectiveness, you should develop the habit of weighing yourself every day after your first morning urine. You should record your weight every day by whatever means (smartphone app or meal diary) and compare the records. You should also be trained to observe and be cautious about how weight changes in response to different types of food. At the same time, you will enjoy seeing an average loss of 150–200 g a day with your own eyes.

One thing to keep in mind is that when someone who is overweight or obese attempts to lose weight, weight loss and blood sugar level reduction will occur at a very fast rate in the beginning. Subsequently, a plateau is reached, at which point, FBS no longer drops readily and weight loss also stalls. There is nothing wrong and there is no reason to be anxious. An important thing to check at this point is hunger. When someone who is used to eating two bowls of rice cuts down to one bowl, the person may feel hunger at first and also lose weight. However, after a certain period, the body adjusts to one bowl of rice. Hunger disappears and weight loss stalls. At that point, the meal size must again be reduced to a half-bowl to overcome the plateau. It is simple but true. The current amount of food intake must be reduced, or the amount must be set one step lower according to the body condition. The absolute amount of food intake must be reduced again by any means including regularly reducing the meal frequency, fasting on one specific day of the week, or fasting every other day.

People sometimes feel shame when they compare the current amount to the amount they used to eat. They will also realize how much they were overeating. Then and only then, food becomes an essential fuel provided by daily meals rather than recreation[99]. Do not mistake this as extreme asceticism. For everything, too much is just as bad

---

[99] Food is fuel, not for fun.

as too little. At the same time, this is the laws of Mother Nature. I hope you can enjoy and be thankful for even the smallest gifts you have been given and enjoy hunger to escape diabetes and recover your health[100].

---

[100] This is a lesson learned after researching the relationship between food and disease and obtaining successful results in clinical practice. The author, who devised the precision diet for diabetes, has long practiced this method and continues to try to always apply it in daily life after escaping from diabetes and metabolic disorder.

11. Do skinny people with type 2 diabetes also need to lose weight?

When skinny people develop wrinkles as they age, they often believe that wrinkles are caused by being too skinny. They become even more concerned about losing weight. At least 90% of type 2 diabetes cases are comorbid with overweight or obesity. How, then, should we view those rare cases of skinny people with type 2 diabetes?

There are two major factors. One is intentional overeating out of fear of losing weight. Instead of gaining weight, they may experience stomach upset and instead lose weight. People who successfully gain weight still appear skinny but their metabolism has gone beyond the normal range. In other words, they may physically appear skinny but experience explosive insulin level increases. The series of processes involved with type 2 diabetes has occurred. Second, they may intentionally consume foods or drugs to help gain weight are not suitable for them, which causes disruptions in their bodies. This could lead to diabetes, which may be accompanied by various symptoms of metabolic syndrome or other chronic diseases.

In these cases, even skinny individuals must lose weight. Their reference weights are those that they maintained for at least 10 years while being skinny and healthy. If the current weight exceeds the reference weight by at least 10%, then the weight goal range for escaping diabetes must be achieved.

12. What about overweight but normal people and skinny people with type 2 diabetes?

The cause of type 2 diabetes is based on a vicious cycle involving hyperglycemia, increased insulin level, and weight gain due to overeating. Most cases are accompanied by overweight or obesity. However, there are rare cases in which a very overweight physique shows normal blood test results. In contrast, very skinny people are sometimes diagnosed with type 2 diabetes or show abnormal markers for various metabolic disorders such as hyperlipidemia. These uncommon occurrences are considered a mystery in the medical community[101].

This is a problem that could be solved by understanding the structural differences between people. A hormone called leptin is secreted mostly by fat; however, inadequate secretion affects the feeding center to cause an insatiable appetite. Affected individuals continue to feel hungry

---

[101] Gina Kolata, a medical reporter from *The New York Times*, wrote an article based on her investigations and interviews of various experts on the processes involved in the efforts to solve this mystery. The article, titled "Skinny and 119 Pounds, but with the Health Hallmarks of Obesity" was published on January 22, 2016. Also refer to additional commentaries in "Skinny Diabetes, Obese Normal" in the author's Current Medical News Commentaries.

despite eating. Continued eating reinforces the vicious cycle of continued hyperglycemia and increased insulin level. People who are born with more fat cells have more room for fat to continue to grow. Despite weight increases and body bloat, their fat grows further still. In such cases, glucose that should be converted to fat to bind to other proteins or free glucose as blood sugar is insufficient. However, beyond a certain point, this condition advances to typical hyperlipidemic and hyperglycemic type 2 diabetes and metabolic disorders. Contrarily, some people are born with less fat. Because they have less fat, they also have less leptin secretion. Accordingly, their appetite continues unabated. Because they have less fat, there have no more fat cells that can grow. Despite maintaining a skinny physique, their blood levels of TG, LDL, and glucose increase, showing hematologic findings typical of type 2 diabetes and metabolic disorders.

Among the classification types used in PDC,[102] Types C or S includes many people who are born with less fat, indicating a high likelihood of skinny diabetes. Types B or

---

[102] Refer to Appendix II

P often includes people born with more fat cells and with normal hematologic findings despite being very overweight or obese. Therefore, the structural differences with which people are born must be understood.

13. How much can you benefit from practicing the precision diet for diabetes? Are there differences in rates of recovery? What are the reasons for these differences?

The keys to the precision diet for diabetes are to identify the appropriate foods for each type of person, determine the amount of food for FMD, and eat regularly by controlling the proportions of vegetables, meat, and grains. When practiced accurately, the benefits appear immediately. It is not magic. Because the cause of type 2 diabetes is various disruptions inside the body due to overeating, this condition can be reversed by stopping overeating. However, in cases with various effects from increased insulin level[103] or that have advanced to micro-

---

[103] Overeating, especially of carbohydrates, causes hyperglycemia due to increased blood glucose level; in response, the level of insulin secreted by the pancreas also increases to cause hyperinsulinemia. Capillary blockage due to repeated inflammation and restoration of the inner vascular walls caused by high blood sugar level could lead to microvascular and/or macrovascular complications. At the same time, increased insulin converts glucose in blood to fat cells, whereby the paradoxical situation of abnormally low blood glucose level is repeated. Therefore, the brain and muscles do not receive a sufficient supply of glucose, which manifests as fatigue, brain fog, thought and concentration disorder, and muscle weakness. Such phenomena appear more frequently or severely when drugs or insulin injection are used. Moreover, this condition may also affect various hormone systems. The feeding center in the brain is disrupted by inhibited leptin secretion by fat cells, which could lead to overeating and even binge eating. This

or macrovascular complications, longer recovery times may be required or recovery may be achieved with some sequelae[104]. In most early cases, speedy complete escape is possible.

FBS and PP2 quickly return to their normal ranges, while morning FBS often remains at high levels during the early stage of the diet or in cases involving severely overweight people. This is because glucose stored as fat inside the

---

condition can also inhibit thyroid hormone, leading to hypothyroidism. By inhibiting cortisol secretion by the adrenal gland, recovery from systemic inflammation is delayed, while inhibition of male and female sex hormones (estrogen/progesterone and testosterone) increases the likelihood of polycystic ovarian syndrome in women and infertility in both men and women. Inhibition of neurotransmitters of the central nervous system, such as serotonin and dopamine, could also cause depression, anxiety, panic disorder, epilepsy, and dementia. It also appears to have a broad range of effects on the immune system and, in particular, inhibits the function of various proteins, including interleukin 6, to interfere with inflammatory response or normal allergic response.

[104] Complete recovery from retinopathy and renal failure, typical microvascular complications, is possible in early-stage disease. Faithfully practicing the precision diet for diabetes does not change the damaged vessels and deformed tissues to new tissues but does stop further damage to the retina and assigns roles to peripheral vessels to achieve functional recovery. Different results may be seen with respect to renal failure based on individual differences and comorbidities; however, in general, individuals with creatinine levels within 3 mg/dL have a high likelihood of complete recovery. Recovery may be difficult at levels higher than that; thus, PDC should be practiced as early as possible. With respect to macrovascular complications, such as cardio- or cerebrovascular disease, much of it is preventive, but if these complications have already occurred, PDC can help to prevent secondary onset. Reversible recovery of remaining sequelae has a low probability and may take much longer.

body is sent to the blood vessels through glyconeogenesis as fasting time increases. The return of FBS to the normal range generally indicates the first signal of escape from diabetes. PP2 is not very reliable since it fluctuates. Subsequently, FBS, body weight, and HbA1c level (once every three months) can be checked to ensure that remission is maintained.

If the precision diet for diabetes is practiced faithfully, no more than 3 months should be enough for cases with HbA1c <10%, while 3–6 months is expected for cases with HbA1c $\geq$ 10%. Differences in recovery times may occur in cases in which different types of drugs were taken for a long time or with comorbid diseases. In particular, anti-diabetic drugs containing sulfonylurea are main culprits of difficulties with escape from diabetes; therefore, discontinuing their use as soon as possible may allow for faster escape.

Generally, the goal should be to maintain an HbA1c level of around 7%, but this target may be adjusted to 7.1–8.5% in elderly people or depending on the situation[105]. The dietary habits should be maintained after achieving the goal, and individuals who have been pricking their finger every day or using continuous glucose monitors (CGMs) do not need to check their blood sugar level any longer. Body weight should be checked daily, while HbA1c level should be checked once every 3 months. If the HbA1c level is stably maintained within the target range for over a year, no other tests are needed, except for checking bodyweight every morning and regular health screening.

---

[105] Refer to "Chapter II-9. What is the target HbA1c value?"

14. What are the short and long-term prognoses of the precision diet for diabetes?

The precision diet for diabetes has a short-term goal of escape from diabetes. Normalization of overweight and hyperlipidemia, which often occur in patients with type 2 diabetes, is an additional secondary benefit. Because blood glucose levels drop quickly to within the normal range, microvascular conditions are recovered, whereby the symptoms that appeared in the retina and kidney dissipate. A rapid decrease in macrovascular burden could contribute significantly to preventing heart and cardiovascular diseases such as stroke.

Elevated insulin level due to hyperglycemia causes direct harm to hormone systems throughout the body. Blood sugar levels drop first and insulin level gradually decreases;[106] as a result, the symptoms also disappear one by one. Overeating and binge eating also begin to disappear as leptin inhibition resolves and hunger dissipates. As the inhibition of cortisol secretion by the adrenal glands is reduced, chronic inflammation is also reduced. As the

---

[106] Normalization is possible within as few as 2–3 weeks.

interfering effect on sex hormone regulation is reduced, maturation of normal eggs occurs to halt the exacerbation of polycystic ovarian syndrome (PCOS), while male sexual dysfunction begins to improve. In addition to self-confidence from improved outer appearance, recovery from depression, anxiety, and panic disorder could be achieved through normalization of neurotransmitters such as serotonin. The diet also contributes to the normalization of levels of immunoproteins, such as interleukin 6, often showing healing of allergies or autoimmune diseases.

In the long-term, the precision diet could help to prevent cancer, which is caused or exacerbated by being overweight, as well as diabetic complications and associated diseases[107].

---

[107] Kyrgios M, Kalliala I, Markozannes G, et al., "Adiposity and cancer at major anatomical sites: umbrella review of the literature", BMJ, 2017;356:j477. This article reviewed over 200 clinical trials on the relationship between adiposity and cancer, finding strong evidence for associations with cancers of the pancreas, kidney, ovary, biliary tract, esophagus, colon and rectum, bone marrow-multiple myeloma, stomach, breast, and endometrium. The results reported in the article, which was widely publicized in *The Guardian*, were selected by the British National Health Service as educational material for national health. Refer to https://www.nhs.uk/news/cancer/wide-range-of-cancers-now-linked-to-being-overweight/

15. Are there enough follow-up cases?

The lengths of the various clinical follow-up cases range between a few months to several decades. Countless people have escaped from diabetes and are living healthy lives while practicing the precision diet for diabetes. With continued introduction of people to this diet, increasing numbers of people are escaping from diabetes. Moreover, more medical institutions are professionally assisting in this escape from diabetes[108].

There is, however, a lack of records and reports. To address this lack, basic work is being carried out to collect follow-up cases and data for dissemination not only in South Korea but also worldwide. Such efforts are expected to soon bear fruit.

Several groups[109] have published data on cases involving complete cure of type 2 diabetes using low-carbohydrate

---

[108] PDC using the professional precision diet for diabetes is offered in nine locations; eight in Seoul, South Korea and one in Toronto, Canada. Many physicians are receiving professional training and planning to implement the program and the number of professional organizations is forecasted to increase. Refer to http://www.ecmclinic.com or http://www.precisiondiabetescare.com

[109] A prime example is Virta Health (USA), with whom Dr. Sarah Hallberg is affiliated. It publishes articles on remission rates and 1-year and 2-year remission

157

diets and fasting or FMD as well as post-cure maintenance cases, although they did not classify people by type. Moreover, a growing number of nutritionist and physician groups[110] are establishing evidence by compiling and analyzing articles comparing calorie-restricted and low-carbohydrate diets and attempting to change the national dietary guidelines. The published reports claim that the long-term observational results of the effects of low-carbohydrate diets demonstrate the need to change national dietary standards or those recommended by medical groups.

---

retention rates for remission achieved by low-carbohydrate diets and online care provided by professional coaches. The study results are accessible to anyone from www.virtahealth.com and webinars are used for continued promotion.

[110] Examples include the British Public Health Collaboration, a team of policymakers from Western Australia, Canadian Clinician for Therapeutic Nutrition (ccfortn.ca), and Dietdoctor from Sweden. In the US, individual physicians and researchers affiliated with universities or research laboratories are publishing results every five years based on their own research findings in an effort to actively declare their opinions and inform the improvement of the dietary guidelines in the US.

16. What are the reasons behind successful and failed cases?

In a world where specific foods and health supplements claiming to be beneficial are increasingly promoted and consumed, it is difficult to accept any aspect of the precision diet for diabetes which is requires choosing foods according to the type of person, extremely reducing the proportion of carbohydrates contrary to conventional dietary guidelines,[111] and claiming the benefits of fasting and FMD. Because these concepts conflict with general knowledge, many people initially reject the method. Despite its amazing health benefits and shortcut to escaping diabetes, many people will not even try the precision diet due to the false perception that it is not trendy and lacks evidence. This is one of the reasons for this guide.

Unlike the early 2000s when low-carbohydrate diets and the fasting or FMD part of the precision diet for diabetes were first devised, these concepts have become

---

[111] Refer to, "To Reverse Type 2 Diabetes, Flip the Food Pyramid Upside Down", Dec. 13, 2017, an article by American endocrinologist Caroline Roberts, MD, who shares the claims that I have been making for a long time.

increasingly better known worldwide, along with studies on the relationship between food and disease. The concepts regarding the different approaches to food for different types of people are difficult to find elsewhere.

Whether through personal experience or propensity, individuals who easily accept something new and try it without bias usually succeed. Of course, those with strong willpower also have a high probability of success. It is unfortunate to find people who have fallen into despair after strictly adhering to existing diabetes dietary guidelines, general dietary guidelines, drug therapy, and insulin injections with almost superhuman willpower. These people often build a mental barrier to accepting something new that is not universally used. Despite this, once they make up their mind to try once again by correcting their misdirected course, many individuals quickly achieve escape from diabetes. This is very fulfilling. What do they have to lose by fasting for several days or changing their diet by drastically reducing the proportion of carbohydrates and eating foods that suit their type?

There is nothing we can do for people who say they will wait until they can understand intellectually or until it becomes universally accepted. We also see people with very weak willpower who are influenced by the words of those around them and information from the Internet. Others do well but suddenly fail due to criticism from someone close to them. There are many failed cases. However, the probability of failure is low among those who diligently check their blood sugar level and take photos of their food. This is because they have already been trained to confirm the relationship between food and values. They get back up even when they fall. Everybody runs experiences plateaus and emotional downturns. That is why continued professional assistance and support communities are needed. While some people become anxious and uncertain about hitting a plateau, many people ultimately succeed in escaping diabetes by following the guidelines. I sincerely hope that everyone can successfully escape from diabetes through the precision diet for diabetes.

17. What options are there to reduce failure?

Unless you have an accurate understanding and strong willpower, it is not easy to succeed on your own. It is not impossible, of course. Because expansive knowledge and experience are essential, professional assistance is necessary in most cases. If possible, receiving professional guidance in real-time from a coach or counselor well-trained in the precision diet for diabetes for at least the first weeks could significantly increase the probability of success. It is also good to use a smartphone to record your condition and to use services that provide real-time counseling and coaching[112]. It may also be necessary to continue to receive assistance and care for management after escaping from diabetes.

It is important to accurately understand this guide before attempting PDC. Because PDC involves completely changing conventional knowledge and lifestyle habits, it will not be easy at first. It takes some time to get used to new lifestyle habits, but this will become a road to

---

[112] As of 2019, a platform for real-time online counseling, care, and training with well-trained specialists (care managers) is being established. It will be introduced and disseminated at http://www.precisiondiabetescare.com.

escaping diabetes, preventing and recovering from diseases, and living a completely healthy life. Even better would be to read this guide over and over to the point of memorizing it. It is also advisable to build basic knowledge through various media platforms such as YouTube and SNS[113]. A better understanding of the medical reasons and guidelines based on the precision diet for diabetes could help reduce failure.

Another good method is to form groups with people who are in similar situations. Online/offline communities to study this guide; share knowledge, information, experiences, and emotions; provide encouragement; and progress together toward the common goal of escape from diabetes could help reduce failure.

---

[113] Refer to the "Precision Diabetes Care" Facebook page and YouTube channel operated by the author. Podcasts by Dietdoctor or Low Carb MD are recommended for English-speaking audiences, although they lack classifications of food according to individual type of person. High-quality information on low-carbohydrate diets and fasting or fasting-mimicking diets from a medical perspective can also be obtained.

18. How long do I have to practice the precision diet for diabetes?

PDC with the precision diet for diabetes as its central pillar involves readjustment of all lifestyle aspects, including diet and exercise. It is not used temporarily to address diabetes, obesity, or metabolic problems followed by a return to an improper lifestyle. Although it is initiated to solve a problem, PDC is the starting point to modify all aspects of life, including diet, exercise, bathing, and breathing, to methods that are most suitable for you. Therefore, learning and practicing PDC as a new lifelong health habit could be a shortcut to escape from diabetes, as well as disease prevention and health promotion. Escape from diabetes itself does not take long. For people with HbA1c <10%, about three months is enough if the precision diet for diabetes is practiced accurately. For people with HbA1c ≥10%, 3–6 months should be enough. Various complications and adverse effects stemming from diabetes also gradually disappear. Although natural aging cannot be stopped, optimal conditions can be maintained. Lifelong light consumption of foods appropriate for your type as part of an appropriate and well-balanced diet are also associated with longevity[114].

---

[114] The topic of longevity is beyond the scope of this guide, but it is an associated long-term effect. Researchers have realized that the experimental and observational results of diets intended to treat diabetes are directly linked to longevity and are introducing them for this purpose. Professor Valter Longo is the director of the Longevity Institute at the University of Southern California. The subtitle of his book, *The Longevity Diet,* is "discover the new science behind stem cell activation and regeneration to slow aging, fight disease, and optimize weight". Light eating is the common point among claims made by various longevity scholars in Japan, which traditionally is a country with the longest life expectancy. Recently, numerous physicians, researchers, and scholars, including Dr. Jason Fung and 2016 Nobel Prize in Physiology or Medicine Laureate Dr. Yoshinori Ohsumi, have provided additional research and clinical findings to support effect.

19. What is the cost-effectiveness of diabetes care with the precision diet for diabetes?

It is very common for people to be prescribed drug therapy for diabetes or prediabetes. On top of the costs associated with drugs and insulin injections, doctor visits, checking and managing HbA1c levels, managing complications (usually in hospitals), and self-monitoring of blood sugar levels the other costs include lost opportunity costs at work and home for such care. Although it is difficult to calculate the exact figure, it is undoubtedly significantly high. Even drug costs alone are significant. In her TED lecture, Dr. Sarah Hallberg cited her research findings[115] that discontinuing drug therapy could save $2,000 per year.

Although each country has different medical systems and methods, a savings of $2,000 each year from drugs alone would result in significant cost-effectiveness, especially in young people. The bigger problem is that spending that much money to adhere to drug therapy could still lead to or even exacerbate complications[116]. The study concluded that

[115] Dr. Sarah Hallberg, Reversing Type 2 diabetes starts with ignoring the guidelines, TEDx Purdue U, "Our analysis showed that our patients could save over $2000 a year just on the diabetes meds they were no longer taking."

even if the cost is invested from the beginning, it cannot prevent complications (or death) that would require even greater costs. Even if it is difficult to calculate the costs, recovering from diabetes and maintaining health may have very different values for people in different economic conditions.

The precision diet for diabetes does not cost anything. Significant cost savings could be achieved with a little bit of study and the will and effort to change your lifestyle. The cost is saved from significantly reducing or completely discontinuing drug therapy, while typical food costs could be halved by fasting or FMD. Even if you consume small amounts of high-quality food that is right for your type, you will still come out ahead. Although economic value is being mentioned, it must be understood that savings in cost and expenditure are bonuses. You should experience this on your own as you keep in mind that the most important thing, which cannot be bought, is a shortcut to escape from

---

[116] Refer to results from clinical trials, including ACCORD, ADVANCE, and VADT. For details, review "Chapter III-6. Can the treatment modalities used in modern medicine effectively prevent complications?"

diabetes, prevention of chronic diseases, and extension of life.

20. Is exercise necessary? If so, what type of exercise is good?

Exercise is not directly associated with diabetes treatment. It has only a transient effect of lowering PP2. Regarding weight loss, exercise is the least cost-effective and generally ineffective[117]. It is impossible to lower FBS or HbA1c by exercise alone. That does not mean exercise is useless. Regarding its importance in PDC, it ranks sixth, following diet (1–5).

Adding exercise to your precision diet for diabetes regimen is certainly desirable. It is also important to differentiate what type of exercise is right for what type of person. The types of exercise that could be helpful for weight loss include aerobic training such as running, hiking, bicycling, and swimming [118]. When exercise time is increased, aerobic training and resistance training have similar effects on weight loss; however, in general, aerobic training is

---

[117] Refer to "Chapter III-9. What are the reasons and scientific evidence to support the treatment of diabetes by dietary therapy alone?"

[118] Willis LH, Slentz CA, Bateman LA, et al., "Effects of aerobic and/or resistance training on body mass and fat mass in overweight or obese adults", J Appl Physiol (1985). 2012;113(12):1831-1837.

more effective for weight loss and control and, thus, for escaping diabetes. The recommended exercise time, based on study results, is three sessions per week with three 25-minute sessions for 75 total minutes per week for strenuous exercise and three 50-minute sessions per week for 150 total minutes of non-strenuous exercise[119]. The type of exercise that is right for you should be selected based on such basic knowledge. Exercise can generally be divided into those which include sweating or no sweating.

Type B individuals should choose exercises that cause significant sweating, including those that cause shortness of breath and rapid heartbeat such as hiking or running. Exercise that prevents sweating, such as swimming, must be avoided. A sauna or hot bath for heavy sweating after exercise or in daily life could be beneficial and warm water should always be consumed during and after exercise and in daily life. Breathing exercises are just as important as physical exercise; the main point is long inhalations. Breathing exercises with four seconds of inhalation, four

[119] Arem H, Moore SC, Patel A, et al., "Leisure time physical activity and mortality: a detailed pooled analysis of the dose-response relationship", JAMA Intern Med., 2015;175(6):959-967.

seconds of hold, and two seconds of exhalation should be repeated, with times increased by the same percentages.

Exercise with heavy sweating is also good for type P individuals. The exercise regimen should focus on the lower extremities, such as running, hiking, and bicycling and the exercises should cause shortness of breath and heavy sweating. Sitting baths that keep the body below the navel warm and make the upper body sweat are good and drinking water should be cold. Breathing exercise should be adjusted to have similar inhalation and exhalation times.

Type C individuals should not sweat heavily. Therefore, they should practice yoga, walking, or swimming, rather than strenuous exercise, and should exercise to sweat as little as possible. When the body is heated after exercise, a cool shower is needed to quickly cool the body surface. No matter how hot the weather, hot water should always be consumed. Breathing exercises should be adjusted to have similar inhalation and exhalation times.

It is also not good for type S individuals to sweat or heat their body surfaces. Swimming is the most ideal exercise, while fast walking in a cool area may be agreeable.

Bathing or showers should be performed with lukewarm or cool water. Water consumed during or after exercise should be room temperature or slightly cooler. Breathing exercises with four seconds of exhalation, four seconds of hold, and two seconds of inhalation should be repeated and trained to have longer exhalation than inhalation times.

While exercise does not have a high priority for the goal of escaping diabetes, adding exercise suitable to your type during the precision diet for diabetes could be helpful for overall health and mood change.

21. Are there tools or methods to effectively managing blood sugar levels and dietary therapy?

Advances in Internet technology and smartphone availability are foreshadowing innovations in various treatment methods and sectors within medicine. Some sectors forecast the near future and prepare for shortcomings, while other sectors have been commercialized and are being utilized. Many novel technologies are now in use for the management of chronic diseases, diabetes, and weight control, while other technologies are being tested and further improved technologies are forecasted. In particular, technological advancements that seamlessly close the gap between patients and physicians or professional counselors are essential and effective for the management of chronic diseases such as diabetes, obesity, and metabolic disorders[120].

---

[120] Michaelides A, Raby C, Wood M, et al., "Weight loss efficacy of a novel mobile Diabetes Prevention Program delivery platform with human coaching", BMJ Open Diabetes Research and Care, 2016;4:e000264.

Michaelides A, Major J, Pienkosz E Jr, Wood M, Kim Y, Toro-Ramos T., "Usefulness of a novel mobile diabetes prevention program delivery platform with human coaching: 65-week observational follow-up", JMIR Mhealth Uhealth, 2018;6(5):e93.

In clinical practice, continued education, practice and management of guidelines through real-time consultation, and effective collection of treatment and consultation records are key for the management of chronic diseases. In particular, real-time consultation and advice from professionals play important roles in supplementing awareness and willpower in the process of achieving an escape for diabetes by changing one's lifestyle and habits using a precision diet for diabetes. A smartphone, which most people use often, could be a good connection tool to send and receive blood sugar levels in real-time via text messages, email, or professional apps, while questions and advice regarding foods and lifestyle interventions could also be provided. For patients or the general public who may find it difficult to remember everything in this guide due to the expansive content, summaries of educational information through mobile apps or YouTube play an important role in achieving the goal of escape from diabetes. From the perspective of physicians or researchers,

Murray E, Daff K, Lavida A, et al., "Evaluation of the digital diabetes prevention programme pilot: uncontrolled mixed-methods study protocol", BMJ Open, 2019;9:e025903.

collecting and publishing data on well-managed and effectively treated cases to build medical evidence is also important. Ultimately, such digital technologies could be very effective ancillary tools to significantly help disease and health management in the general public, even though they cannot replace the experience and determinations of medical professionals.

Epilogue

The academic field of medicine deals mostly with science. The term "mostly" reflects the multitude of additional variables to consider in the human body other than those addressed by basic laboratory science. The term also applies to other fields such as the physiological applications of chemistry, biochemistry, and physics. It also applies to changes such as abandoning calorie count, which was previously considered common sense; eggs considered bad one day to a complete food the next; and aspirin being a useful tool to prevent heart disease to a harmful drug that should be avoided. The blame lies on the fact that medicine is based on science, which is based on great uncertainties. Putting aside the confusion among the general public, even medical professionals are divided by different opinions and claims. This is the reason why differences among people must be studied.

Medical training in college is often based on memorizing a significant amount of information. There is no choice since a large volume of data needs to be inputted into the brain, including the structures and functions of the human body as well as different diseases and their treatment. The problem surfaces in clinical practice in which actual patients are being cared for. The time from passing the national medical license examination, when the confidence as a physician is at its highest, to being placed in real-world clinical settings is very short. Medical practice based on memorized information and established guidelines is often useless in actual clinical settings. Because of this disparity, some professionals take the extreme choice of leaving the field that they worked so hard to get into or transfer to a different field.

Clinical practice is often referred to as a form of art. While some people who perform honorably and successfully, others abandon their conscience and approach medicine as just an occupation. Based on my lengthy experience in teaching medical students and other doctors, the likelihood of success is higher in those who are creative in applying and integrating their basic medical knowledge while diligently observing the clinical setting.

The global perception of diabetes is problematic. The discovery and subsequent fear of type 1 diabetes may have been transposed to type 2 diabetes. The time has come to break free from this perception. These conditions should be viewed from completely different angles. While I previously fought on the frontline of clinical practice and such trends, I now take comfort in hearing similar voices worldwide. Fortunately, aggressive efforts in western societies in the past 5 years have researched the relationships between diseases and foods to reduce or discontinue drug therapy and change the medical guidelines. Studies on the background reasons and explanations of the mechanisms involved are pouring out from the field of diabetes and metabolic disorders. It is fascinating to see my claims over the past two decades, which could not be expressed properly in English as it is not my native language, now being expressed in English worldwide by western physicians. It makes me slightly jealous but it is desirable in the bigger context.

This guide organizes my claims about diabetes, obesity, and metabolic disorders in a question-and-answer format and attempts to demonstrate that nearly identical claims are being made worldwide. While evidence confirmed by textbooks or clinical trials is still lacking, this guide attempts to account for treatment processes and situations in real-world clinical practice that have been or will be introduced in articles.

I consider it my responsibility to continue to introduce new updates or findings. Even if my efforts are not recognized, it is my mission to persevere if it helps to eradicate diseases and help patients.

I dream about a day that this guide can start with experience of few people who escaped from diabetes to becoming a shortcut to eradicating diabetes for millions of people around the world. IGIT

Appendix I: New proposal for the disease classification of diabetes

This disease started from the term diabetes, short for diabetes mellitus, based on the concept of excess sugar in urine. However, it is becoming increasingly evident that a new disease classification is needed as we learn more about the true nature of this disease. Diabetes itself has been classified into type 1, type 2, gestational, and other specific types, while new classifications are being added and some subtypes of type 2 diabetes are showing similar characteristics to those of type 1. Diabetes was previously classified as pediatric or adult but this method of classification has already lost its validity and is rarely used. Another reason for the need to reclassify diabetes is the fact that it occurs in conjunction with a series of metabolic disorders. The author was the first in the world to advocate the need for a new classification and establishment of disease concept that considers a series of metabolic disorders, including obesity, diabetes, hypertriglyceridemia, and hypercholesterolemia; associated complications including direct microvascular/macrovascular complications caused by hyperglycemia as well as indirect complications involving the hormone, autonomic, and immune systems caused by hyperglycemia-induced hyperinsulinemia; and situations with no or limited insulin secretion due to autoimmune disease or drug abuse. The most reasonable method may be to recategorize type 1, type 2, and other diabetes as hyperglycemic hyperinsulinemia, and hyperglycemic hypoinsulinemia, respectively.

I. Hyperglycemic hyperinsulinemia

1. Causes: Hyperglycemia due to overeating and binge eating, especially continued overeating of meals with high proportions of carbohydrates

2. Symptoms and complications;

1-1) Symptoms of hyperglycemia: increased thirst, frequent urination, blurred vision, frequent infections, and slow-healing sores.

1-2) Microvascular complications: retinopathy, renal failure, tingling and numbness in hands and feet, cold sensitivity, Buerger's disease, etc. Macrovascular complications: hypertension, heart failure, angina pectoris, stroke, etc.

2) Symptoms of hyperglycemic hyperinsulinemia visceral complications: fatty liver, obesity, hypertriglyceridemia, hypercholesterolemia, type 2 diabetes, gestational diabetes, idiopathic diabetes, hepatitis, etc.

3) Hyperinsulinemia symptoms (hormonal complications): hunger, overeating, binge eating (leptin inhibition); depression, anxiety, panic disorder, insomnia, dementia (inhibition of CNS neurotransmitters, such as serotonin and dopamine); hypothyroidism (thyroid hormone inhibition); severe type 2 diabetes or type 1 diabetes (pancreatic hormone inhibition, pancreatic failure, and pancreatic cancer); impaired recovery from inflammation and immunosuppression (inhibition of adrenal hormone cortisol); menstrual irregularity, PCOS, and infertility (inhibition of female hormones); hyposexuality, erectile dysfunction, and infertility (male hormone inhibition);

increased allergic inflammatory response and autoimmune disease (interleukin 6 inhibition)

3. Treatment:

1) Precision diet for diabetes: periodic fasting (PF) or periodic fasting-mimicking diet (PFMD) with a personalized, precision low-GI/GL diet

2) Complications: symptomatic treatment

4. Commentary on treatment mechanisms: precision diet for diabetes → decreased glucose → decreased insulin → increased sympathetic tone and decreased hormone control → increased metabolism and decreased thyroid, pancreatic, adrenal, and sexual hormone control → normalized levels

5. Application: while not absolute, types B and P have a higher probability of hyperglycemic hyperinsulinemia; because they are of vagotonia (parasympathicotonia) types,

the precision diet for diabetes often shows much more effective results.

II. Hyperglycemic hypoinsulinemia

1. Causes: congenital, autoimmune disease, drug-related (long-term use of drugs containing sulfonylurea for type 2 diabetes), pancreatic destruction due to cancer or surgery, unknown.

2. Symptoms and complications

1) Symptoms of hyperglycemia: increased thirst, frequent urination, blurred vision, frequent infections, slow-healing sores, etc.

2) Symptoms of hypoinsulinemia: extreme hunger; unintended weight loss; irritability and other mood changes, including hypersensitivity and anxiety; fatigue and weakness; etc.

3. Treatment: insulin injection + precision diet for diabetes - PF or PFMD with a personalized, precision low-GI/GL diet

4. Commentary on treatment mechanism: increased insulin + precision diet for diabetes → Decreased metabolism and increased parasympathetic tone → decreased extreme hunger → increased weight and decreased fatigue, normalized irritability and other mood changes

5. Application: while not absolute, types C and S have a higher probability of hyperglycemic hypoinsulinemia; because they are of sympathicotonia type, the combination of insulin injection and precision diet for diabetes on a limited basis may be beneficial.

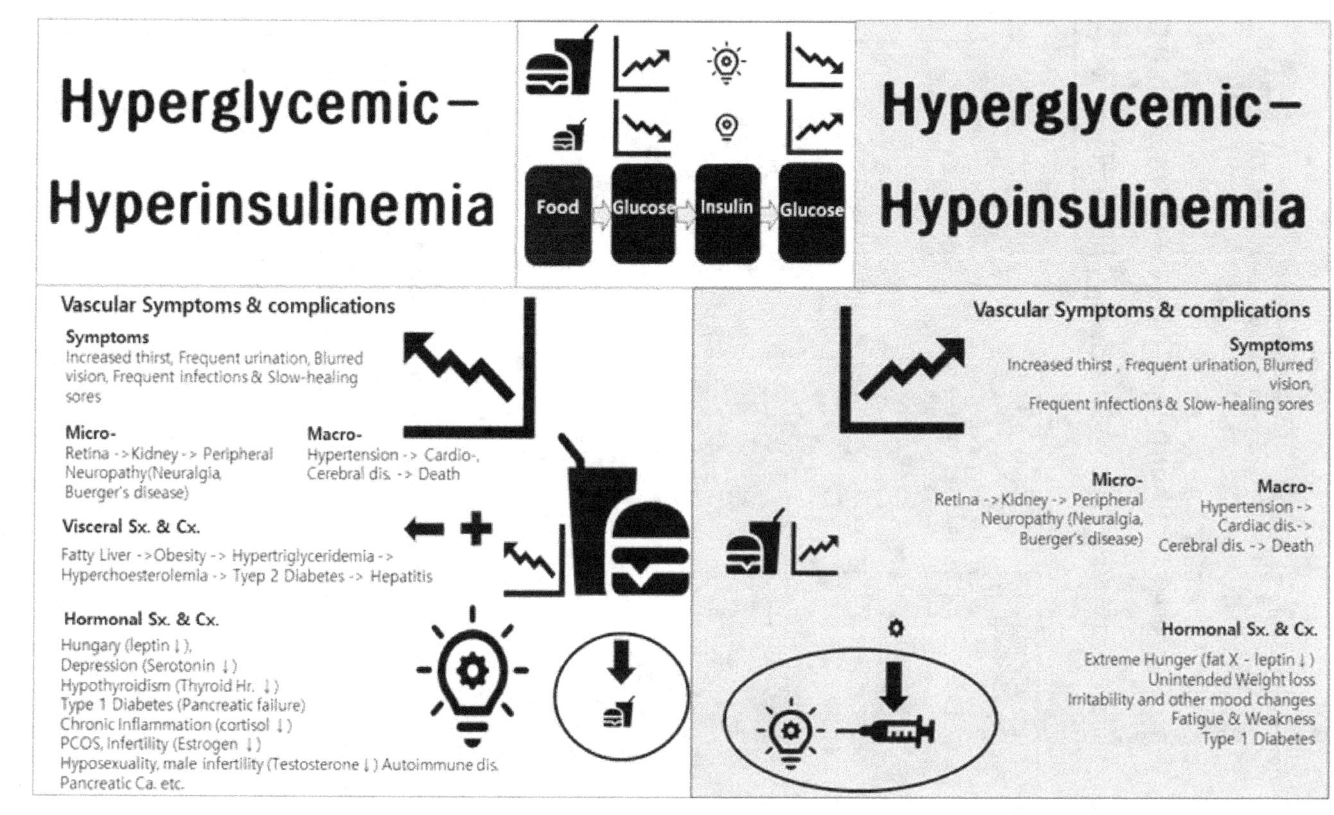

Hyperglycemic –
Hyperinsulinemia

Food Glucose Insulin Glucose

Hyperglycemic –
Hypoinsulinemia

Vascular Symptoms & complications

Symptoms
Increased thirst, Frequent urination, Blurred vision, Frequent infections & Slow-healing sores

Micro-
Retina -> Kidney -> Peripheral Neuropathy(Neuralgia, Buerger's disease)

Macro-
Hypertension -> Cardio-, Cerebral dis. -> Death

Visceral Sx. & Cx.
Fatty Liver -> Obesity -> Hypertriglyceridemia -> Hyperchoesterolemia -> Tyep 2 Diabetes -> Hepatitis

Hormonal Sx. & Cx.
Hungary (leptin ↓),
Depression (Serotonin ↓)
Hypothyroidism (Thyroid Hr. ↓)
Type 1 Diabetes (Pancreatic failure)
Chronic Inflammation (cortisol ↓)
PCOS, Infertility (Estrogen ↓)
Hyposexuality, male infertility (Testosterone ↓) Autoimmune dis.
Pancreatic Ca. etc.

Vascular Symptoms & complications

Symptoms
Increased thirst , Frequent urination, Blurred vision,
Frequent infections & Slow-healing sores

Micro-
Retina -> Kidney -> Peripheral Neuropathy (Neuralgia, Buerger's disease)

Macro-
Hypertension -> Cardiac dis.-> Cerebral dis. -> Death

Hormonal Sx. & Cx.
Extreme Hunger (fat X - leptin ↓)
Unintended Weight loss
Irritability and other mood changes
Fatigue & Weakness
Type 1 Diabetes

Appendix II: Examples of diet and weekly meal plans by types

Type B(Beef)

How to Eat –Diet Precision low-carb diet & PF(PFMD)

1. **Light eating** – Regular light eating(must feel hungry
   at least 30 -60 minutes before the next meal)
2. **Regular meals** – Set mealtimes(1,2,3,,,)
3. **Meals with appropriate proportions** – vegetable-meat-grain(refer to figure below)

Vegetable	Meat	Grain

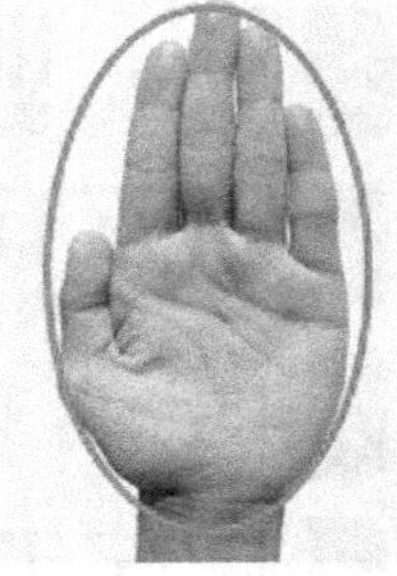 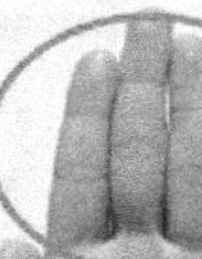 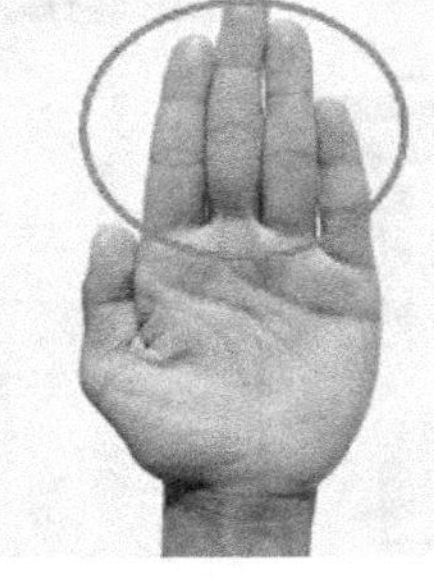 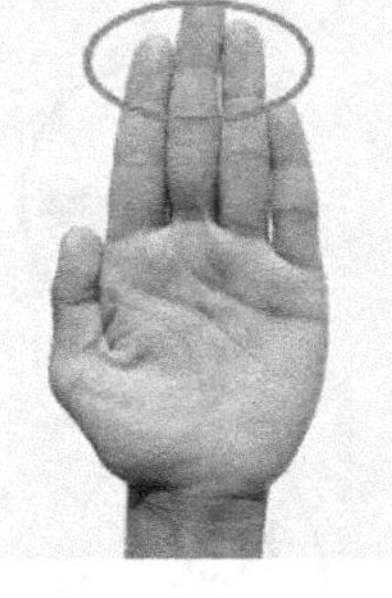

Radish, Carrot, Lotus Root, Beet, Taro Burdock, Pumpkin, Zucchini, Eggplant, Bean sprout, Mushroom, Onion, Tomato, Avocado	Beef, Chicken & Poultry, Duck, Pork, Lamb, Goat, Eggs, Milk(Cow/Soy), Cheese, Butter, Beans & Peas, Legumes, Nuts, and Tofu / Oils(Canola, Soy, Corn, Sesame, Perilla)	Rice(White/Brown), Wheat flour-based foods(bread, pasta, noodles, etc.), Oat, Corn, Potato, Yam ***Beverage** : Coffee(hot, 1 cup a day), Hot water

How to Exercise **Perspiring**(Running, Bicycling, Mountain climbing, Hiking etc. 3 times or more a week)
Bathing(Sauna or Hot Bath) /**Breathing**(Long inhalations)

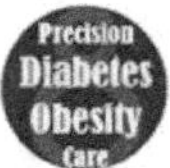 316-4750 Yonge St., Toronto, M2N 0J6, ON, Canada
precisiondiabetescare@gmail.com
www.precisiondiabetescare.com 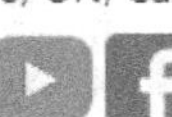 "Precision Diabetes Care"

Type B : 7-Day Meal Plan

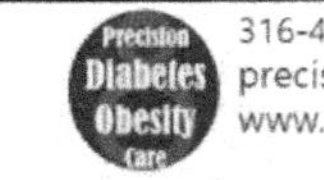

* Could be applied or modified according to preferences or situations

Day 1	Day 2	Day 3	Day 4	Day 5	Day 6	Day 7
Breakfast	**Breakfast**	**Breakfast**	**Breakfast**	**Breakfast**	**Breakfast**	**Breakfast**
Beef omelet	Fried tofu	Fried eggs	Cheese omelet	Boiled eggs	Vegetable omelet (Onion, Bell pepper)	Omelet cake (oinions, carrots)
Coffee(warm)	Black Tea	Milk(warm)	Milk(warm)	Coffee(warm)	Black tea	Milk(warm)
Drinks*	**Drinks**	**Drinks**	**Drinks**	**Drinks**	**Drinks**	**Drinks**
Hot water or Black Tea	Hot water or Black Tea	Hot water or Black Tea	Hot water or Black Tea	Hot water or Black Tea	Hot water or Black Tea	Hot water or Black Tea
Early dinner	**Early dinner**	**Early dinner**	**Early dinner**	**Early dinner**	**Early dinner**	**Early dinner**
Chicken salad** (Bell pepper, Onion, Radish, Beet, Tomato etc)	Beef salad (Bell pepper, Onion, Radish, Beet, Tomato etc)	Tofu & Fried Onion, carrot	Chicken salad (Bell pepper, Onion, Radish, Beet, Tomato etc)	Beef salad (Bell pepper, Onion, Radish, Beet, Tomato etc)	Tofu & Fried Onion, carrot	Beef steak & Roasted garlic, mushroom

* To alleviate hunger

**For people with gastrointestinal disturbance, all foods, including meats and vegetables, must be cooked

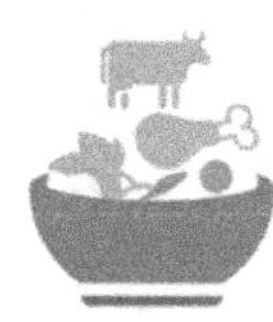 316-4750 Yonge St., Toronto, M2N 0J6, ON, Canada
precisiondiabetescare@gmail.com
www.precisiondiabetescare.com  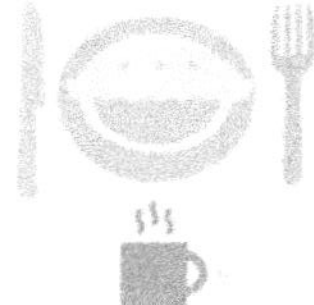 "Precision Diabetes Care"

Type P(Pork)

How to Eat –Diet | **Precision low-carb diet & PF(PFMD)**

1. **Light eating** – Regular light eating(must feel hungry
   at least 30 -60 minutes before the next meal)
2. **Regular meals** – Set mealtimes(1,2,3,,,)
3. **Meals with appropriate proportions** – vegetable-meat-
   grain(refer to figure below)

Vegetable	**Meat**	**Grain**
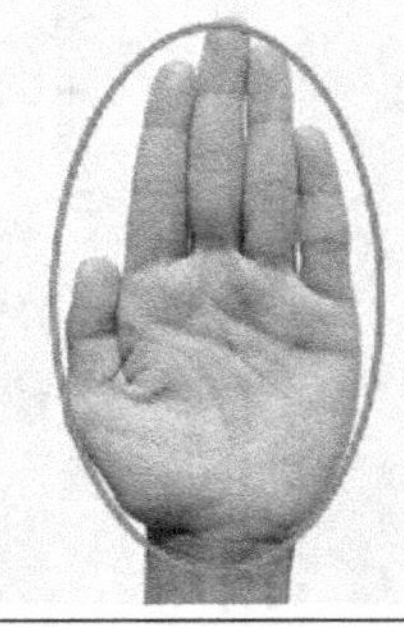	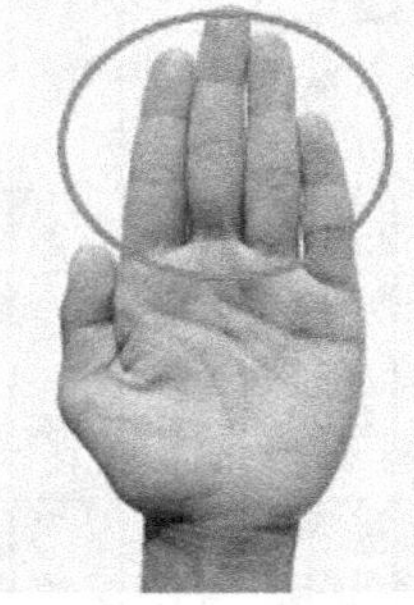	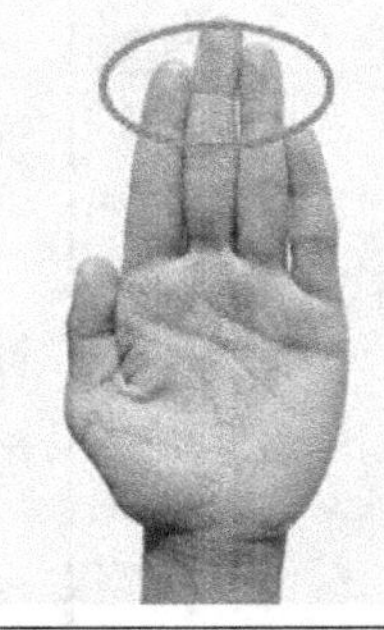
Radish, Carrot, Lotus Root, Lettuce, Cabbage, Cucumber, Water Dropworth, Bok choy, Brussels sprouts, Broccoili, Cauliflower, Bean sprout, Pumpkin, Zucchini, Mushroom, Avocado	Pork, Beef, Eggs, Milk(Cow/Soy), Cheese, Butter, Fish, Seafood(shrimp, crab, clams, squid etc.) Beans & Peas, Nuts, Tofu	Rice(White), Barely, Buckwheat, Wheat flour-base foods(bread & Pasta, noodles, etc.) Oats, Rye ***Beverage** : Coffee(cold, 1 cup a day), Cold barley tea or water, Green tea

How to Exercise | **Perspiring**(Running, Bicycling, Mountain climbing, Hiking etc. 3 times or more a week)
Bathing(Sauna or Hot Bath) /**Breathing**(Similar inhalation and exhalation)

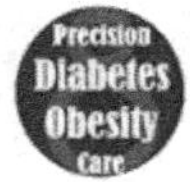

316-4750 Yonge St., Toronto, M2N 0J6, ON, Canada
precisiondiabetescare@gmail.com
www.precisiondiabetescare.com 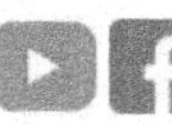 **"Precision Diabetes Care"**

Type P : 7-Day Meal Plan

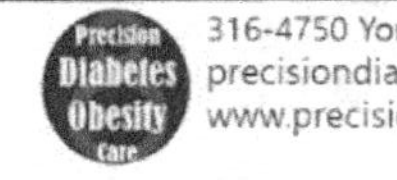

* Could be applied or modified according to preferences or situations

Day 1	Day 2	Day 3	Day 4	Day 5	Day 6	Day 7
Breakfast	**Breakfast**	**Breakfast**	**Breakfast**	**Breakfast**	**Breakfast**	**Breakfast**
Bacon omelet	Boiled Tofu	Fried eggs	Cheese omelet	Boiled eggs	Vegetabel omelet (Broccoli, Cauliflower, Cabbage)	Bacon omelet cake
Green Tea	Milk(lukewarm)	Milk(lukewarm)	Green Tea	Milk(lukewarm)	Green Tea	Iced Coffee
Drinks*	**Drinks**	**Drinks**	**Drinks**	**Drinks**	**Drinks**	**Drinks**
Cold water or Barley tea	Cold water or Barley tea	Cold water or Barley tea	Cold water or Barley tea	Cold water or Barley tea	Cold water or Barley tea	Cold water or Barley tea
Early dinner	**Early dinner**	**Early dinner**	**Early dinner**	**Early dinner**	**Early dinner**	**Early dinner**
Pork salad** (spring mix, cucumber)	Beef salad (spring mix, cucumber)	Tofu & Steamed cabbage	Pork salad (spring mix, cucumber)	Seafood(cod) salad (spring mix, cucumber)	Seafood(scallop) salad (spring mix, cucumber)	Pork rib steak & Roasted garlic, mushroom

* To alleviate hunger

**For people with gastrointestinal disturbance, all foods, including meats and vegetables, must be cooked

316-4750 Yonge St., Toronto, M2N 0J6, ON, Canada
precisiondiabetescare@gmail.com
www.precisiondiabetescare.com
"Precision Diabetes Care"

Type C(Chicken)

How to Eat –Diet | **Precision low-carb diet & PF(PFMD)**

1. **Light eating** – Regular light eating(must feel hungry
at least 30 -60 minutes before the next meal)
2. **Regular meals** – Set mealtimes(1,2,3,,,)
3. **Meals with appropriate proportions** – vegetable-meat-
grain(refer to figure below)

Vegetable	Meat	Grain

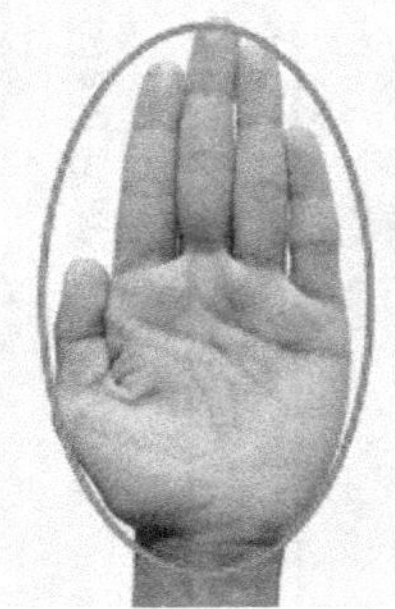 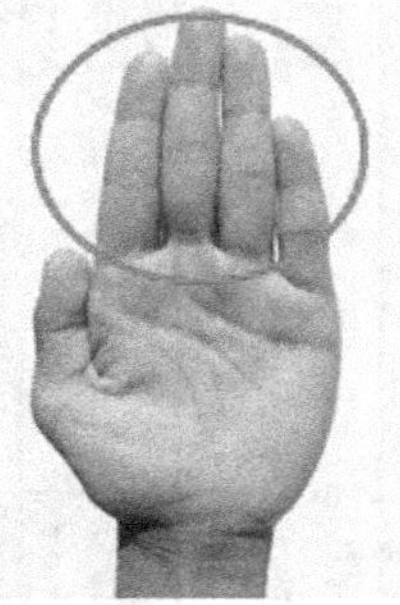 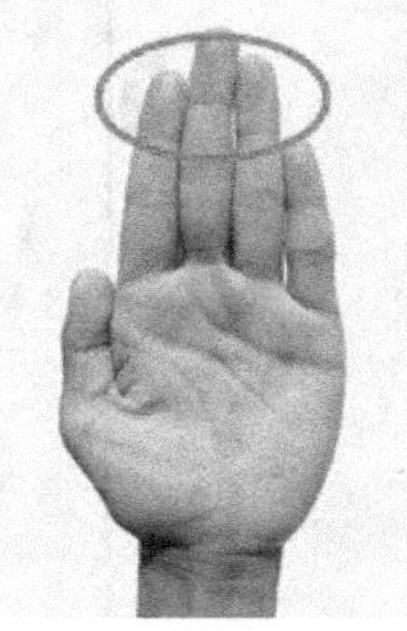

Seaweeds(dried seaweed, brown seaweed, and tangleweed, Nori, Onion, Green Onion, Spinach, Chives, Bell pepper, Paprika, Bean sprout, Pumpkin, Zucchini, Eggplant, Tomato, Radish, Carrot, Taro, Burdock	Chicken & Poultry(duck, turkey), Lamb, Goat, Beef, Eggs, Beans(Soy, Kidney)& Pea, Nuts, Tofu / Oils(Sesame, Soy, Corn, Canola)	Rice(Brown, Glutinous, White), Corn, Potato, Yam, Millet ***Beverage** : Tea(Honey, Ginseng, Ginger, Japanese Apricot, Lemon, Date, Jujube), Hot water.

How to Exercise **Non-perspiring**(swimming and yoga at least three times or more a week)

Bathing(Lukewarm or cold bath) /**Breathing**(Similar inhalation and exhalation)

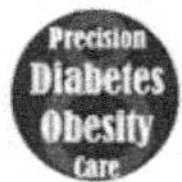 316-4750 Yonge St., Toronto, M2N 0J6, ON, Canada
precisiondiabetescare@gmail.com
www.precisiondiabetescare.com 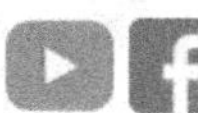 **"Precision Diabetes Care"**

Type C : 7-Day Meal Plan

* Could be applied or modified according to preferences or situations

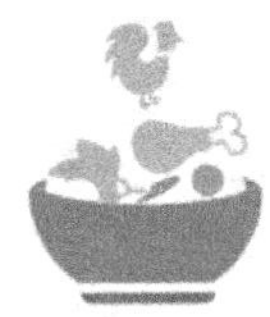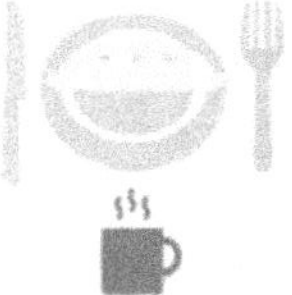

Day 1	Day 2	Day 3	Day 4	Day 5	Day 6	Day 7
Breakfast	**Breakfast**	**Breakfast**	**Breakfast**	**Breakfast**	**Breakfast**	**Breakfast**
Chicken Omelet Ginger tea(hot)	Fried Tofu Ginger tea(hot)	Fried egg Milk(warm)	Cheese Omelet Milk(warm)	Poached egg Ginger tea(hot)	Veg. Omelet (Onion, Bell pepper) Ginger tea(hot)	Pepper, Onion Omelet Cake Milk(warm)
Drinks*	**Drinks**	**Drinks**	**Drinks**	**Drinks**	**Drinks**	**Drinks**
Hot water or Tea(Ginseng, Date)	Hot water or Tea(Ginseng, Date)	Hot water or Tea(Ginseng, Date)	Hot water or Tea(Ginseng, Date)	Hot water or Tea(Ginseng, Date)	Hot water or Tea(Ginseng, Date)	Hot water or Tea(Ginseng, Date)
Early Dinner	**Early Dinner**	**Early Dinner**	**Early Dinner**	**Early Dinner**	**Early Dinner**	**Early Dinner**
Chicken Salad** (Bell pepper, Onion, Tomato etc)	Chcken & Fried Onion, carrot	Tofu & Fried Onion, carrot	Beef Salad (Bell pepper, Onion, Tomato etc)	Chcken & Fried Onion, carrot	Tofu & Fried Onion, carrot	Fried Chicken & Pickled Radish

* To alleviate hunger

**For people with gastrointestinal disturbance, all foods, including meats and vegetables, must be cooked

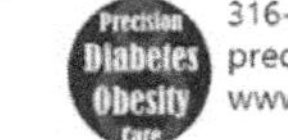

316-4750 Yonge St., Toronto, M2N 0J6, ON, Canada
precisiondiabetescare@gmail.com
www.precisiondiabetescare.com

"Precision Diabetes Care"

Type S(Seafood)

| **How to Eat –Diet** | **Precision low-carb diet & PF(PFMD)** |

1. **Light eating** – Regular light eating(must feel hungry
   at least 30 -60 minutes before the next meal)
2. **Regular meals** – Set mealtimes(1,2,3,,,)
3. **Meals with appropriate proportions** – vegetable-meat-
   grain(refer to figure below)

Vegetable	Meat	Grain
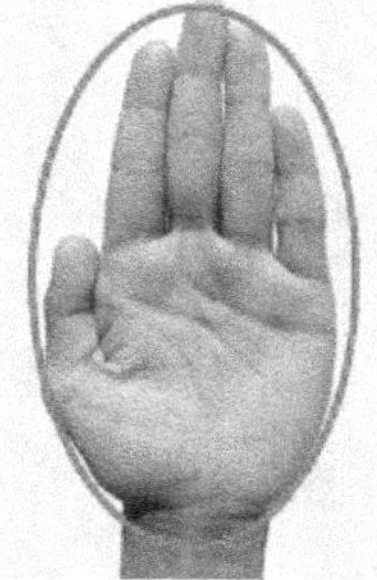	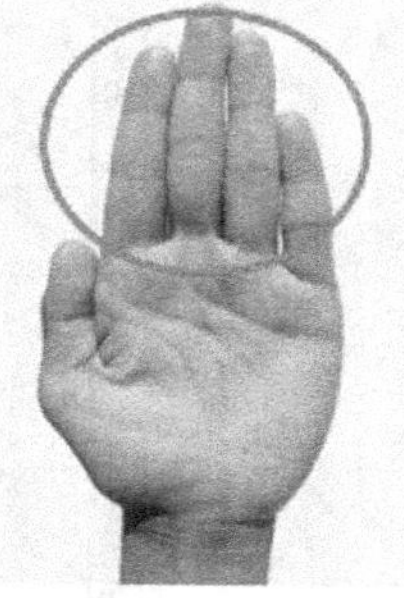	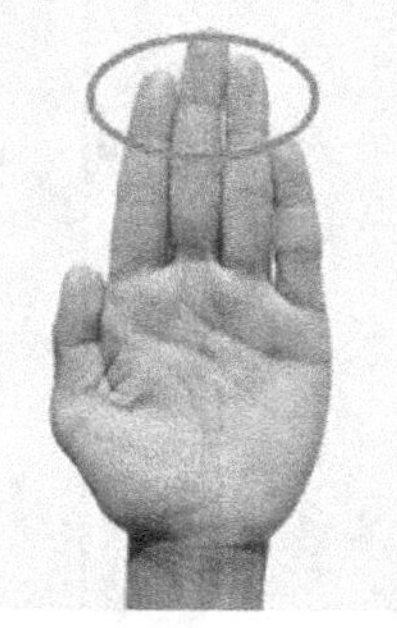
Lettuce, Cabbage, Cucumber, Water Dropworth, Bok choy, Brussels sprouts, Broccoili, Cauliflower, Mungbean sprout, Zucchini, Nori(dried seasweed), most green leafy vegetables.	Saltwater fish(haddock, halibut, sole, cod, sea bream, sea bass, mackerel, etc.), Clams, Mussel, Scallop, Oyster, Shrimp, Crab, Lobster, Squid, Octopus, Egg White, Red bean, Mung bean, Tofu	Rice(White), Buckwheat, Millet, Rye ***Beverage :** Tea(buckwheat, quince, lukewarm), Cold water

| **How to Exercise** | **Non-perspiring**(swimming and yoga at least 3 times or more a week) |

Bathing(lukewarm and cold bath) /**Breathing**(Long exhalations)

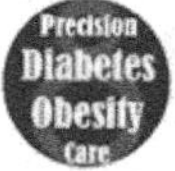 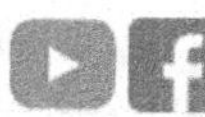
316-4750 Yonge St., Toronto, M2N 0J6, ON, Canada
precisiondiabetescare@gmail.com
www.precisiondiabetescare.com   **"Precision Diabetes Care"**

Type S : 7-Day Meal Plan

* Could be applied or modified according to preferences or situations

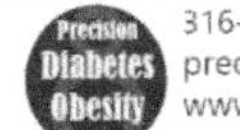

Day 1	Day 2	Day 3	Day 4	Day 5	Day 6	Day 7
Breakfast	Breakfast	Breakfast	Breakfast	Breakfast	Breakfast	Breakfast
Crabmeat Omelet Water	Veg. Omelet (Broccoli, Cauliflower, Cabbage) Buckwheat tea	Fried egg Water	Seafood Omelet(clam, fish meat) Buckwheat tea	Boiled egg Water	Veg. Omelet (Broccoli, Cauliflower, Cabbage) Buckwheat tea	Seafood(clam, fish, crab meat) Omelet Cake Buckwheat tea
Drinks*	Drinks	Drinks	Drinks	Drinks	Drinks	Drinks
Water or Buckwheat tea	Water or Buckwheat tea	Water or Buckwheat tea	Water or Buckwheat tea	Water or Buckwheat tea	Water or Buckwheat tea	Water or Buckwheat tea
Early Dinner	Early Dinner	Early Dinner	Early Dinner	Early Dinner	Early Dinner	Early Dinner
Cod Salad** (spring mix, cucumber)	Scallop Salad (spring mix, cucumber)	Tofu & Steamed Cabbage	Fish(Haddock) Salad (spring mix, cucumber)	Fish(Salmon) Salad (spring mix, cucumber)	Tofu & Steamed Cabbage	Lobster & Broccoli, Cauliflower, Cabbage

* To alleviate hunger

**For people with gastrointestinal disturbance, all foods, including meats and vegetables, must be cooked

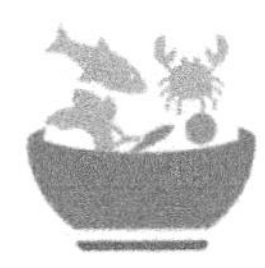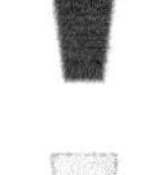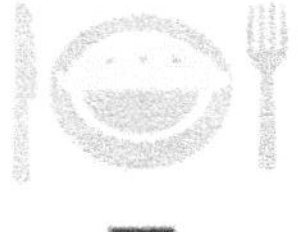

316-4750 Yonge St., Toronto, M2N 0J6, ON, Canada
precisiondiabetescare@gmail.com
www.precisiondiabetescare.com

"Precision Diabetes Care"

">